What's in This Book

In the pages that follow, renowned holistic doctor and nutrition-ist Bernard Jensen, Ph.D., speaks from the heart on a trio of life's most intimately connected—yet widely misunderstood—topics: love, sex, and nutrition.

As one of the founding fathers of the modern natural health movement, Dr. Jensen has been instrumental in helping thousands of people overcome their health problems. As a leading clinical nutritionist, he has developed special diets and exercise programs for a multitude of health problems. Now, for the first time, he explains the significant relationship between food and the emo-tional self. Does what we choose to eat affect our love lives? Do these choices shape our relationships? Is there a natural way to enhance sexual potency? The answer is a resounding, "yes." And, inside, Dr. Jensen tells us why.

His account is chock-full of personal anectdotes, tips, and tid-bits culled from 57 years as a health counselor, worldwide trav-eler, and student of cultures from every age and location. Dr. Jensen imparts his level-headed lessons with warmth and wisdom. No quick fix, here. But those ready to take the time to open their minds to his simple and practical principles will be on their way to healthier, happier, and—yes—sexier lives!

Be good to your self physically, mentally, spiritually.

Dr. Bernard Jensen

To Marie, my loving and faithful partner
through many struggles, blessings,
and journeys in life.

LOVE, SEX & NUTRITION

Dr. Bernard Jensen

AVERY PUBLISHING GROUP INC.
Garden City Park, New York

The medical and health procedures in this book are based on the training, personal experiences, and research of the author. Because each person and situation is unique, the editor and the publisher urge the reader to check with a qualified health professional before using any procedure where there is any question as to its appropriateness.

The publisher does not advocate the use of any particular diet and exercise program, but believes the information presented in this book should be available to the public. If you have a history of back troubles, or other physical restrictions, we recommend that you consult with your health care provider before beginning any exercise program.

Because there is always some risk involved, the author and publisher are not responsible for any adverse effects or consequences resulting from the use of any of the suggestions, preparations, or procedures in this book. Please do not use the book if you are unwilling to assume the risk. Feel free to consult a physician or other qualified health professional. It is a sign of wisdom, not cowardice, to seek a second or third opinion.

Cover design by: Martin Hochberg and Rudy Shur
Cover photo by: FourByFive, Inc.
In-house editor: Nancy Marks Papritz
Typesetting by: Multifacit Graphics, Inc.

Library of Congress Cataloging-in-Publication Data

Jensen, Bernard, 1908-
    Love, sex, and nutrition.

    Includes index.
    1. Sex--Nutritional aspects. 2. Sex (Biology)
--Nutritional aspects. I. Title.
QP251.J458 1988   613.9'6   88-8124
ISBN 0-89529-395-1.

Printed in the United States of America

10 9 8 7 6 5 4 3 2 1

Contents

PART FOUR: PUTTING IT ALL TOGETHER

Preface

Close your eyes for a moment and imagine that you and your mate are two separate stars whirling through space. You each have an identity and an orbit to travel within throughout life. But you are also very close in time and space. As you grow closer still in your love, each is attracted to the other by magnetic forces. These forces cause you to begin to revolve about each other. Finally, you combine to form a double star. At times you remain apart from each other in your journey through the heavens. But you are never too far from the magnetic attraction that binds you. Gradually—as the revolutions continue—you are united again. True, you and your companion are different. But to an observer, your double star will always appear to be one. And the love-shine created by your fusion will be truly spectacular to behold.

When a love relationship is right, two bodies, two minds, and two spirits fuse in harmonious love. Because men and women love differently, their coming together, like the fusion of stars, is sometimes difficult and always a challenge. Each must meet the needs of the other, yet discover completion and fulfillment in the other. It is precisely because this loving relationship is such a challenge that each individual must be prepared; each must be healthy and strong in body, mind, and spirit. This is because, like the brilliant light from the double star, a wonderful, satisfying love is the result of combining our forces. The first step towards creating that light is our decision to try.

Do you really want to have a more wonderful love life? Do you consider yourself a good lover and do you understand the basic anatomy and workings of the sexual system? Are you really healthy or do many of those nagging little "bugs" always seem to keep you under the weather? Does job-related stress prevent you from being happy? Do you realize that in a literal sense you are what you eat, and that if you're eating mainly high-sugar, high-sodium, high-cholesterol, and low-fiber foods that you are slowly but surely poisoning yourself? Do you understand the intimate relationship between nutrition and sex? Are you willing to examine your strengths and weaknesses honestly, with a desire to improve the quality of your life?

If you sincerely desire to improve your love and sex life and your emotional and physical health, then I want to help.

I find it ironic that no three subjects have been discussed at greater length—yet understood less—than love, sex, and nutrition. Love is the subject of numerous books, television talk shows, and—in a general sense—forms the basis of the plots of most movies and TV soap operas. Human sexuality has been more thoroughly researched, analyzed, and written about in the past twenty years than in all of recorded history. And as for nutrition, it would appear that everyone, including doctors, athletes, movie stars, models, and even military leaders, has unveiled a secret diet plan guaranteeing health, beauty, and a wonderful love life.

So, you ask, why produce another book on these subjects? There are at least three reasons. One, though the popularity of these sex manuals, love treatises, and nutrition guides is indisputable, I doubt that there has ever been a time or place when there remains more confusion, unhappiness, disappointment, and overall distress over these important areas of our lives. We need to comprehend the complex forces at work within us and within society before we can hope to improve our lots. This book addresses these forces.

Two, though much has been written about these subjects separately, almost never will you see love, sex, and nutrition discussed in the same context. This is unfortunate because, as we will learn, the three are inextricably linked—so much so, that to consider one without the others is illogical and leads to many wrong conclusions. Perhaps because I have followed the path of natural healing, my approach to these problems has been different from that of most health-care professionals, sociologists, psychologists, and other experts.

Three, my search for solutions to problems associated with love and sex was based on practical, everyday experiences rather than on laboratory research or textbook studies. I was stimulated by my patients' questions regarding their most common and intimate problems. Frankly, I did not know many of the answers. I went scurrying to find out, first looking into my own life. I questioned and listened to people who seemed to have happy, lasting relationships. I visited countries around the world. In the process, I made many false starts and drew many mistaken conclusions. But in the end I learned. And what I learned I present here. I hope it will help you to discover and create a beautiful, healthy lifestyle for yourself and for your lover.

Several years ago, I discovered a simple truth: There is no such "creature" as a love problem, sex problem, or nutrition problem that can be treated symptomatically. Mental and physical problems are intimately linked. Without an understanding of the interrelation of body and mind, we may treat symptoms as ends in themselves, not as the warnings of body/mind/spirit imbalance that Nature intended them to be.

We must therefore begin to treat the human being as a whole. When the whole person maintains healthfulness—body, mind, and spirit—health problems disappear. This truth is so simple that many of us refuse to accept its wisdom. As a result, I am afraid that most of us search entire lifetimes for the missing ingredients without realizing we carry them within us all the time.

When we stop to think about it, not only are love, sex, and nutrition closely interrelated, they are surrounded and influenced by a host of social, ethical, and moral conditions, interrelated and producing symptoms of their own. We live in a time of great technological and cultural change, a time of debilitating stress and anxiety for many people. Our working, eating, and living patterns have altered drastically in the past thirty years. Most of us are constantly on the go, snatching food and rest whenever and wherever possible with little regard for the cumulative effects on our health. Moral standards have changed dramatically over the last several decades, also, leaving many of us unsure of where to find an anchor in a sea of spiritual upheaval. Is it any surprise, then, that under such conditions we would find an increase in the love, sex, and nutrition problems in our society?

In the 1980s, it seems we read or hear about a significant medical breakthrough almost every day. Modern medical science continues to find new techniques for treating diseased hearts, new drugs for patients with various cancers, new ways to perform successful organ transplants. Indeed, we have taken huge steps in treating some human illnesses. Nevertheless, we remain far removed from finding "cures" for most cancers, heart disease, and many infectious diseases. Chronic diseases and the drugs used to treat them, are having an increasingly profound effect on our daily lives as well. As we see many of these types of diseases on the increase, requiring larger and larger doses of drugs to which our bodies have become immune, we must each ask the question, "Where is the healthy and happy life that I thought was to be mine?"

Though science can cure many modern maladies, only we can control the healthfulness of our daily lives. Medical treatments that rely on drugs and surgery have very little bearing on this so-called better health that most of us in Western societies have come to expect. It is true that we have a longer life expectancy than did our ancestors, but this is chiefly because of the lowered death rates among infants and children made possible after most childhood infectious diseases were eradicated earlier in this century. Indeed, such averages as "life expectancy" can be quite misleading. As individual adults, we have gained little in increased years. Ironically, with all our progress, much about us remains unchanged. The life expectancy of a 45-year-old today is only a few years longer than that of a 45-year-old in 1887.

This book is therefore based on the premise that we are fooling ourselves if we believe that our "progressive" civilization, with its technological achievements and "advanced" medical techniques, guarantees us good health, good sex, or good anything. Perhaps our first admission must be that even the "experts" have much to learn regarding love and sex. Only recently, for example, have scientists begun to discover the relationships between diet and disease, and between various diseases and sex. What we do understand is that these areas of human existence are too important to ignore, to leave to misunderstanding, or to relegate to graffiti-language explanations on restroom walls.

Yes, modern technology and new medical techniques have provided us with the opportunity to secure better foods, better sex, better health, generally better lives. But a key ingredient remains obscured. Increasingly we are finding evidence that the external environment is not the answer, that no matter how much technology "improves" our foods, medicines, surgical techniques, and the host of other contemporary assistance we receive—it is not enough. The answers must lie somewhere else.

The conclusion to which a great deal of contemporary scientific evidence points is one basically akin to the conclusion that great thinkers have reached since time began: More than anything else, the way we see and know ourselves, our attitudes towards ourselves and others, determines our success or failure. We cannot be successful lovers until we first understand and love ourselves. We cannot be healthy unless we first have healthy attitudes towards our own bodies and minds.

Love, sex, and nutrition are interdependent. What we eat and otherwise put into our bodies affects our mental attitudes, emotions, and physical health. Diet can influence whether we are physically active or sedentary, radiant and clear-complected or sallow. Similarly, as we shall see, all of the chemical processes of love and sexuality are directly controlled by the chemicals we ingest. (Although we might not like to think in terms of "eating" chemicals, that's exactly what we do.) Thus, if we really want wonderful love lives, one of the very first steps we must take is to understand the potential effects of what we put into our bodies.

Just as what we eat affects our love lives and overall health, love and sexuality (or the lack of either) can determine our attitudes—whether we are depressed or happy, nervous or relaxed, and almost every other aspect of our beings. Being "lovesick" is not just a state of mind that afflicts adolescents. Love and sex even influence what we eat and, if we are particularly upset by a love relationship, we may go so far as to ignore eating altogether. The destructive cycle of poor nutrition contributing to a negative mental attitude and low self-image promote a poor love- and sex life. However, once we develop and maintain loving, healthy attitudes, and learn the secrets of good nutrition, our diets will nourish our immune systems, and we will find that diseases pass us by. This knowledge is my chief gift to you in this book. Distilled to its basic elements, the message is clear: You—and only you—hold the power to control your own destiny. You can determine the success or failure of your sex and love life; your physical, mental, and spiritual health; and almost every other aspect of your life. I hope to serve as your guide.

In the following pages I share with you a practical, living philosophy of love and sex that focuses on a union of the body, mind, and spirit in one healthy being. If you are searching for answers based on exhaustive research in some sterile laboratory, or if you are looking for easy answers, then you have come to the wrong place. Any insights I offer have evolved both through years of introspection and through working with people just like you.

I have deliberately avoided highly-technical language wherever possible, and the few technical terms that do exist—such as terms for glands and hormones—are less important than what they stand for. This reflects my belief that you need to know that various endocrine glands secrete hormones with a direct impact on your sex life, as well as how some of these hormones work; but you don't need to be concerned about specific names.

I am not interested here in quizzing your knowledge about human anatomy and physiology. Neither am I promoting my philosophy of life. My purpose is to share ideas that have worked for me and thousands of other people just like you. The principles explained here, if practiced diligently and sincerely, are guaranteed to make you a better lover, better friend, better and healthier person. The test is the measure of your life, and only you can determine your success.

So let us go then, you and I, on a journey to wonderful love, pleasurable sex, and glorious health.

Introduction

If you truly want a wonderful love life and you are willing to work for it, I believe you can have it.

During my past fifty years of work as a clinical nutritionist I have counseled thousands of patients. As a result, I believe beyond the shadow of a doubt that love and health are so closely knit together that changing the level of one alters the level of the other. I have never met a person who could say, "I feel wonderful," who did not also have a healthy, harmonious "love life"— that is, a positive, loving attitude toward others—whether or not it included an active sex life or a current romantic attachment.

We are each created to give and receive love. This is our natural heritage. When we are not giving or receiving love in a balanced, harmonious, natural way, deficiencies occur in our innermost being. These deficiencies reveal themselves through many symptoms—depression, loneliness, destructive relationships, weight problems, bitterness, inferiority feelings, workaholism, alcoholism, drug abuse, a critical spirit, violence, sexual abnormalities, and many other forms. Most doctors, psychiatrists, and psychologists treat only these symptoms. I believe we must treat the whole person on the other end of the symptom.

My success in the natural healing art is due to a remarkable truth I discovered many years ago: The doctor does not heal. Nature heals. Sometimes, however, Nature can use a helping hand. My approach to healing is based on finding the best way to provide Nature with that helping hand. Proper nutrition can help Nature to get things started.

As a nutritionist, I feel there are foods for the spirit, soul, and body, and all three must be fed before we can lead happy, fulfilled lives. As you will learn in Part One of this book, love feeds all three levels. Love is whole, pure, and natural food. Love is a healer, a lifter, a joy food. It should be a regular part of your diet.

Because sex is one of the highest and most fulfilling expressions of love, it will be discussed at some length in Part Two of this book. And, because the fullest, most satisfying expressions of love and sex require a foundation of good health, I have dedicated Part Three to the subject of nutrition. "Putting It All Together" is the title of Part Four—and it is designed to help you do just that.

With this book, my role is to help you find the right path for your life, to point you in the right direction. Your role is to recognize and acknowledge your own hidden needs as you follow the direction I've indicated.

Together, we are going to explore many varieties of experience in the chapters that follow. This is because each individual is unique—and the same problem in two different people may require two entirely different approaches. Therefore, the key is to know yourself, to become a best friend to yourself, and to resolve to meet the needs you encounter as faithfully as possible.

I want you to consider my advice as you would walk through a flower garden. Some of the flowers in this garden are meant for you; the rest are meant for others. Pick those that you recognize as yours, and leave the others as you journey through love, sex, and nutrition.

Part One
LOVE

Chapter One
Love Conquers All?

Love should be joyful, a continuous celebration between two people who join their hearts, minds, and bodies together. Living as closely as lovers do has great blessings and great lessons for both individuals. As a result, the experiences of love can be a great source of wisdom. Surely, one of life's greatest privileges is being intimately involved in observing and assisting our lovers as they develop their gifts, talents, and abilities. Equally rewarding is the love and support our lovers give us, thereby helping us to develop our own gifts to a greater level than we might on our own.

The traditional social-moral ideal of love and marriage in this country is that young people remain chaste, complete their formal education, choose a partner, and then take wedding vows. These vows include maintaining the marriage bond, "for better or for worse, in sickness and in health, until death. . . ." In this traditional concept of marriage, fidelity is considered an integral aspect, as are courage and fortitude to stand by a spouse and to work through all difficulties and obstacles encountered throughout life.

However, traditions change. And, thanks to a myriad of social, cultural, and economic upheavals, much of this tradition has been topsy-turvy for the past few decades. If it is inherent in the nature of man to love—and I believe it is—we therefore need a refresher course on what love is and what love is not.

FALSE LOVE

Almost all of us have experienced love at one time or another or, if we have not, we have spent a great deal of time dreaming about love and the "ideal" relationship. It's hard not to in our society.

The cliché image of love popularized in movies, music, TV, and romantic fiction portrays a glamorous woman swept away by a handsome man to live happily ever after in a world free of hard work, anxiety, stress, or other common problems. If disagreements or troubles do occur, they are always minor and disappear with a flurry of kisses and sexual intimacy within the brief time segment required to watch the show or read the chapter. Luckily, most of us are realistic enough to be able to admit that love is both more—and less—than this distorted Hollywood image that beckons to us from every direction we turn.

Our conception of love usually forms during our youthful years. A bumper sticker on a teenager's car that passed me recently pronounced, "Life is a beach." As we grow older, many of us forget the carefree zest for life that grabbed us when we were teenagers such as that bumper sticker expressed. Yet it is important to remember that the teen years mark the formation of most of our attitudes, particularly those towards love and sex. If our love values were distorted when we were young, there should be little surprise when our love relationships disintegrate later in life.

For example, some young people have been taught that the body and sexual feelings are somehow unnatural, worthless, or something to overcome. Such beliefs tend to approve the spiritual nature of man while disapproving or denying the physical nature. I have met people who are afraid to enjoy and appreciate their bodies and normal sexual feelings because of such beliefs. I don't believe there is any benefit or truth in assuming that God disapproves of our bodies, man and woman, or of sexuality, or, for that matter, of any of the other physical functions. I believe that we are meant to live in a constant state of joy and love for our bodies and respect and love for the vitality of other human beings.

We are created, on the physical level, to be sexual beings. We are designed, on the emotional level, to take pleasure in our sexuality. We are intended, on the spiritual level, to love. And love, when understood correctly and maturely, assures that pleasure and sexuality will be expressed with both freedom and responsibility.

Love, pleasure, and sexuality are inherent aspects of our human nature. They are meant to be expressed in our lives. However, modern life can distract us from the true, natural expressions of love. As a result, it takes a certain amount of wisdom to have a healthy love life on this planet.

LOVE VS. PLEASURE

Pleasure, not love, is the greatest motivating factor at work in our culture today. Indeed, the easiest way to become a millionaire in today's world is to develop some novel form of pleasure, advertise it, and market it widely. It is ironic that in our culture, people spend a lot of money on pleasure, many not realizing that they are destroying the beauty of their bodies, their health, and their lives in the process.

If we really loved and respected our bodies, we would not abuse them with drugs and alcohol. We would not stuff them with processed foods laced with chemical additives. We would not soak our lungs with tar and nicotine, let our muscles get flabby from lack of exercise, or punish our hearts with fat-loaded diets.

We are killing our bodies by a combination of neglect, ignorance, and poor choices. Though our culture does not "force" us to make poor choices, it does create an atmosphere in which we are strongly encouraged to make poor choices. We are like wide-eyed children on Christmas morning, looking at all the presents under the Christmas tree. It's very hard to resist opening a beautifully wrapped present, even though we know that what's inside might do us more harm than good.

Our culture has become a "Christmas-every-day" culture, and we're buying it, despite the fact that, in our hearts, we know we are ruining our bodies, our minds, and our lives. And it's affecting our sexuality and reproductive systems in obvious and negative ways.

PHYSICAL SELF IMAGE

One of modern culture's biggest misrepresentations is that each of us should be an ideal physical specimen. Although it is important to attain healthfulness, we must accept certain physical limitations if we are to be truly happy.

Our bodies are the only bodies we will ever have. We might as well learn to love them. They may not be perfect—but no one has a perfect body. We must accept the fact that the body comes with the person. We aren't going to be comfortable loving or liking another person if we don't decide to love or like the body that comes with him or her.

But to love another, we must first love ourselves. Why is this? It is more enjoyable to love another person if we first love and

accept our own bodies. If we are worried about how we look all
the time, we won't really be able to accept the love of someone
else, because we won't believe we are "loveable." This can result
in all sorts of ridiculous (though quite real) problems. We won't
trust the person who says, "You're beautiful tonight," or "You're
very handsome," because we won't feel beautiful or handsome.
Our very lack of trust in the other person's feelings about us gets
in the way of our own love for that person because no one can
fully love someone they don't trust. It's a double-bind, a built-in
failure.

So, if you're a woman—give it up. Look in the mirror and say,
"I am beautiful." Do it five or ten times a day if you have to—until
you believe it.

If you're a man, the same thing goes for you. Learn to love that
face and body of yours. Look in the mirror and practice telling the
truth. "I am handsome." You're going to love how you feel when
you believe it.

LOVE AND SEX

Once we accept ourselves, we are ready to begin to understand
love. We often think of love as originating in and flowing from
our soul or mind, while sex is entirely a body-related event or
biological urge. Indeed, people talk about "good sex," just as they
would talk about a "good dinner"! (Sex therapist Dr. Virginia
Masters notes other parallels between love and sex: they share the
same vocabulary, create social bonds, and reflect social change.)
Those of us who view love for the mind and sex for the body are
not alone. It's easy to see how these conclusions can be draw in
our society.

But, while we recognize some truth in this type of categoriza-
tion, we must admit that the relationship between love and sex is
a bit more complex. There can be no love, no sex, until something
moves in the mind. Love and sex both originate from a wonderful
little electromagnetic spark that awakens the love consciousness
or arouses sexual interest. What our minds are like depends upon
our genetic inheritance and our home life, education, relationships, and other experiences.

Love requires kindness, thoughtfulness, and sensitivity to
needs other than the sexual. And these are all mental things. It is
interesting to me that scientists have found a sex center in the
brain—but not a love center. Love is not a physical, biological, or

even primarily emotional process. It involves many parts of the brain and the rest of the body.

Sex has a biological urgency built into it that is driven by the urge for procreation, the survival of man. Love is equally as powerful a drive as sex, but it is a softer one, less urgent, more enveloping and constant. Love is more social, sex is more private. Sex is more like an arrow; love, more like a warm cloud through which the arrow travels.

Considering its relative importance in marriage, I would rate sex at 10 percent. But that 10 percent must be 100 percent for a marriage to be happy, healthy, and fulfilling. This is because if the sex life in marriage is right, many other aspects of the marriage will be positively affected. Conversely, if the sex life in marriage is not right, then many other aspects of the marriage will suffer. The two are intimately linked. We therefore conclude that sex, while pleasurable on its own, is more fully gratifying when it is wrapped in a package of love.

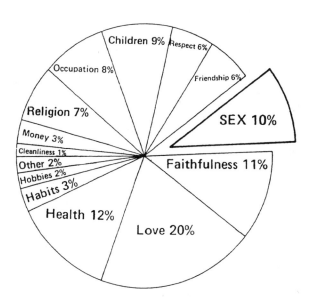

Priorities in Marriage. The percentages selected for each subject category on the chart are, by necessity, somewhat subjective, perhaps a little different for each person and each marriage. But, just as every slice is a part of the whole pie, it takes all the right ingredients to make a good marriage.

REAL LOVE

The New Testament teaches that, "Love is patient and kind, never jealous, never boastful or conceited. Love is never rude or selfish; it does not take offense. Love takes no pleasure in other people's sins or mistakes, but delights in the truth. Love is always ready to forgive, to trust, to hope, to endure whatever life brings."

This wonderful picture of true love is in sharp contrast to the impulsive, sensual, narrow view of love presented in many of today's books, magazines, films, and television programs. It is not true love to look primarily for qualities in another person that would gratify one's own pleasure, ambitions, and expectations. This is because love is first spiritual, something that touches our lives and faith. Second, it is mental—requiring respect, honor, pride, honesty. Only last is true love physical. The outcome of the physical relationship, in true love, depends on a combination of both the mental and spiritual being. Though the spiritual law says what we give comes back to us and we reap what we sow, it is best to consider this law outside the context of true love. For true love exists without expecting anything in return.

It is unfortunate, therefore, that many people say, "If you'll love me first, I'll love you." What we reveal with this statement is our fear of being vulnerable, of being open, of being hurt. We are afraid if we say, "I love you," that the other person will say, "Well, I don't love you." Sure rejection hurts. But unless we learn to take chances and live with vulnerability, we will never be able to fully express real love.

Chapter Two
The Chemistry of Love

These days, we often hear people say, "We're really getting along great—the chemistry is right!" Or, we hear, "They are getting a divorce. The chemistry just wasn't right." Doctors talk about blood chemistry, and nutritionists talk about chemical imbalances in the body. We recognize that there is both a mental and a physical side to "chemistry" in the way that people talk about it, and, as far as human experience is concerned, physical and mental chemistry in life are intimately related.

The chemical processes that go on in our bodies are vitally important in determining the quality of our love lives and our relationships with others—not to mention the level of our health. We can be "high" on love or we can feel "low" when a love relationship has broken up or isn't going well. Scientists tell us that these mental states most definitely are related to changes in body chemistry.

WE LIVE IN A DRUG AND CHEMICAL AGE

We can only begin to understand love, sex, and nutrition by recognizing what scientists have already proven: our blood chemistry affects our moods and personalities. Second, we must admit that never in the history of man have so many chemicals and drugs found their way into our bloodstream—from prescription and over-the-counter drugs to the thousands of chemical additives used in foods. Chemical pollutants from air, water, pesticide residues on foods, and chemicals in the workplace contribute further. Possibly the three most widely-used drugs in this country are alcohol, caffeine, and nicotine—and all three are recognized to be mood-altering drugs that interfere with normal sexual functioning with long-term use. We shouldn't forget *internal* sources of chemical imbalance, either, such as those caused by an unbalanced diet, stress, and constipation. Even fatigue, or strong emotions like anger and jealousy can produce nerve acids that upset the blood chemistry.

It is time that we recognized that our love lives will never be normal until we steer our lives out of the drug and chemical flood that threatens to drown our civilization. We're all looking for a "quick fix" to solve our love and sex problems. However, our best hope is to turn to a "slow fix": a right way of living and a more natural lifestyle.

THE MENTAL CHEMISTRY OF LOVE

What is love, in terms of mental chemistry? One family therapist said, "If my pulse races, that's love . . . an overpoweringly tender feeling toward someone . . . an electromagnetic response or a genuine emotion." This definition might just as well fit the effects of certain drugs on our minds, except for a single, interesting phrase—"an electromagnetic response."

When we get right down to it, all chemistry—whether in a test tube or the human brain—involves "an electromagnetic response," an interaction of electrical and magnetic forces that changes our physical chemistry. We are vibrant beings, influenced by color, music, aromas, tastes, and direct physical contact. When we fall in love, we are interacting electromagnetically with another human being. What we need to realize is that this electromagnetic interaction is not normal when so many unnatural chemicals are influencing what goes on in our brains.

The difference between people and laboratory chemical reactions is that people are free to work out some of the "chemical reactions" by how they choose to respond to each other in various circumstances. We have the power within us to determine our own moods, whether we feel happy, or sad and depressed. We can also control our love lives. Of all the creatures on this planet, only human beings are capable of resolving their differences and creating a harmonious relationship in which each brings out the best in the other.

Condemnation and anger, in this context, are choices we make that are destructive to the natural chemistry of relationships. Destructive emotions are most often found in unhealthy people using unhealthy diets and living unhealthy lifestyles. We can do better if we choose a higher path in life—the path toward whole, pure, and natural living.

In the human brain is a small area called the hypothalamus which acts as a central switchboard, receiving nerve messages from the thinking part of the brain, the emotional centers of the brain, and from all the organs, glands, and tissues of the body. The hypothalamus monitors nearly everything that is going on in the body, including chemistry. This part of the brain also responds to what is going on by triggering nerve impulses aimed at protecting and balancing body functions. The sex center, which initiates processes that influence endocrine gland functions in the body, is located in the hypothalamus.

The mind must be harmonious and balanced before the body chemistry is balanced. We can't live in anger, fear, regret, resistance, and resentment and still expect our body chemistry to be right. Remember, every thought we think touches every cell in our body. In order for "the chemistry of love" to be right in our bodies, the chemistry of love must be right in our minds. What does this mean in practical terms?

We need to love, care for, and nurture our partners. We need to have the right attitude toward them and stay free from blame and criticism. We need to encourage their personal growth, let them be who they are, and know when to leave them alone. Our partners should feel that they are free to be who they really are with us. Change yourself before considering how to change the other person. Be an example for your mates, then they will change themselves. Body chemistry responds to the good we give to our mates, and the chemistry of love begins to harmonize on the physical and mental levels for both partners.

THE CHEMISTRY OF MOODS

In recent years, researchers have discovered many things about the way foods and drugs alter our moods. For example, niacin deficiency can bring about depression, and so can food allergies, low blood sugar, or an underactive thyroid (in some cases due to iodine deficiency in the diet).

Brain chemicals called endorphins have been found to relieve pain and generate a feeling of happiness. They can even produce a natural "high" that is much better than the drugs some people use. Hormones released by various endocrine glands may trigger general excitement, a sense of well-being, sexual arousal, and alertness. These hormones can even influence the metabolism (energy level) upward or downward.

For years, doctors have used drugs like Valium or amphetamines to alter the moods of their patients. Drugs are used to treat depression, schizophrenia, violent tendencies, and other psychological problems. While little is known about how these drugs work, they definitely alter moods effectively. But they are unnecessary for most people.

Since our emotions play a large role in what we call "falling in love," we should realize that what we eat, drink, or ingest can seriously affect our love life by altering our body chemistry which in turn alters our emotions.

CUES TO AWAKENING LOVE

Studies of animals have brought out some interesting facts about the release of brain- and glandular chemicals that are associated with various stages of mating behavior.

One of these facts is that not only reptiles and birds, but also mammals—including humans—are influenced in the initial mating process by odors. Substances called pheromones, released from certain parts of the body, appear to be detected by the hypothalamus of the brain and activate interest in the sex center. For unknown reasons, this process is selective. Not all males and females are drawn to one another. Experiments by a group of West German scientists, for example, showed that blindfolded men and women could identify the perspiration of their mates. Perhaps there is an intuitive knowledge, planted deep within us, that recognizes a compatible mate by odor. This may be the chemical precursor to the development of what we know as love.

Visual cues in humans also play a strong role in partner selection. But experience has shown that this is not a reliable way of identifying a compatible mate. We may like what we see, but we don't see beneath the surface to the real person. Sounds can play a role in mate selection, also. Male birds of many species attract mates by their songs, which are also designed to warn the other males to stay out of their territories. Some male animals make sounds at mating time to attract females. Men and women find certain tones and voice rhythms attractive to the opposite sex. People of many cultures use music to create a romantic environment, and we find that sound plays a role in sexual attraction and stimulation.

This evidence helps us to conclude that our five senses are definitely involved in courtship, mate selection, and family life, triggering the release of hormones and brain chemicals related to sexual behavior and the rearing of offspring. Studies of socialization in higher animals provide evidence that learned behavior is also very important. We can interpret this data to mean higher animals, including humans, need good role models.

LOVE ADDICTION

What can we say, then, about famous lovers such as Don Juan, Casanova, and Cleopatra? Did their body chemistries go haywire? Some theorists say yes.

One current theory proposes that certain people, driven to one love affair after another, are "love-aholics"—addicted to love. Their love addiction is similar to others' addiction to alcohol or cocaine. Researchers now believe that the initial "rush" of falling in love may be due to a combination of hormones and brain chemicals that triggers an emotional "high." Love-aholics are people in love with love, not with other people. They are looking for a chemical "fix" from their own brain and glands, not for someone to settle down and share life with. One Californian, for example, got into the *Guinness Book of World Records* by marrying twenty-six times. "I fall in love, out of love, and back in love again," he said. But is this really love? I think you'll agree with me that this kind of temporary infatuation is superficial and selfish. People who are "in love with love" do not gain the pure joy that results from knowing another person intimately, from sharing their lives with another human being. I recognize that those who repeatedly marry and divorce may have severe personality problems. Body chemistry is not everything. But personality problems tend to create an unbalanced body chemistry sooner or later.

Perhaps the "love addiction" we discuss here stems from a chemical imbalance in the body or from a love-deprived childhood, leading to an abnormal love starvation later in life. The problem may be triggered by nutritional deficiencies or a genetic disorder that leads to a compulsive love "behavior" that never quite succeeds in fulfilling the hidden hunger. The glandular hormones and brain endorphins released during a brief but intense love affair temporarily substitute for what is actually a chemical deficiency, emotional deficiency, or both.

Doctors at the New York State Psychiatric Institute claim that falling suddenly in love is caused by a rapid increase in the brain of a natural chemical called phenylethylamine. The natural high produced is interpreted by the brain as "being in love" and can be quite addictive. The breakup of an intense love affair may be similar to amphetamine withdrawal because of a sudden drop in brain levels of phenylethylamine. This, scientists say, is what results in the classic "broken heart" syndrome. It isn't known what causes levels of the chemical to rise or fall. (People in this state frequently crave chocolate, which is high in phenylethylamine.)

At the opposite end of the scale, a study at Johns Hopkins University in Baltimore focused on investigating a group of patients who were unable to experience intense romantic passion. The problem was traced to a pituitary gland malfunction early in life. The patients formed normal friendships, and some of them married for companionship, but none were capable of that heart-pounding, stomach-sinking delight that most normal people at least occasionally encounter when they fall in love.

Yet another form of love addiction has been investigated by Robin Norwood, a family therapist in Santa Barbara, California, and author of *Women Who Love Too Much*. Women who have experienced parental neglect or abuse, who grew up around bitter family disputes or alcoholic parents, seem to be vulnerable to obsessive love. Many of these women fall in love with men who abuse or neglect them. By doing so, they reproduce the same pattern of rejection they experienced as children. They are unhappily married to unloving men—and deliberately so. The questions posed by Norwood's book have contributed to the discussion of love addiction. Is there a tendency in people to reproduce their childhood emotional experience of home life when they become adults? Is there a chemical basis to this problem, in the functioning of the brain and glands? Perhaps future research will bring us answers to these questions.

LOVE AND HEALTH

As human beings, we are caught in a fascinating "love circle." Unless we are healthy, we can't express truly wholesome love, and unless we love, we can't truly be healthy.

We were all made to give and receive love. There are no physical, mental, or spiritual substitutes for the kind of sharing, caring love that most of us recognize as "real" love. Chronic emotional pain due to a mistaken choice in love partners is not healthy, nor is it justifiable on moral grounds. We have to face such problems realistically and get professional help if and when we need it. We need to do this not only for our mental health. The growing body of medical evidence proves we must do it for our physical health, as well.

In recent years, scientists have looked into the relationship between emotions and the immune system. They found that people who were happy or happily in love had much stronger defenses against disease than those who were depressed or unhappy. They traced the cause of this difference to a relationship between the human nervous system and the immune system.

Somehow, by means of chemical transmitters, our nerves are able to "communicate" how we feel to our immune system, and the immune system is weakened or strengthened accordingly. Without doubt, our attitudes and general emotional state can affect our health. This is yet another reason why we need to work

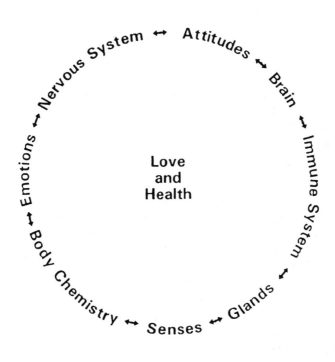

The Circle of Love

at developing healthy, happy love relationships. What goes into our minds affects our immune system, our natural defense against disease.

Harvard University researchers have found that not only self-less love and caring for others, but also a sense of humor and lack of cynicism, are linked to good health. Incredible as it seems, this Harvard team reported that by remembering or visualizing times of loving or being loved for as little as one hour, the level of the immune response was raised temporarily.

Remember that our moods have a powerful effect on the glands that release chemical transmitters to various cells throughout the body. A depressed state often reinforces a negative, unwillingness to fight in the immune system, but good humor and elation can marshal the positive chemical forces of the body to ward off the strongest of attackers. More than one "miracle cure" has turned out to be nothing more, and nothing less, than the positive attitude of a person determined to overcome any obstacle.

BECOMING A HEALTHY LOVER

Realizing that we live in a world where pollution, perversion, violence, and disease are constantly around us, what can we do to become healthy lovers? How are we to cope with the drug and chemical flood of our time? How can we have healthy families and healthy children in a world where power, money, and success are given higher priority than love and healthy human relation-ships? We can begin by resolving to become healthy lovers. Here are some tips to get you started.

- Make a lifestyle checklist of healthy and unhealthy habits and behavior. Then, begin to eliminate the unhealthy factors. We have to stop breaking down before we can build ourselves up. Include critical attitudes and negative talk on your list. If you are married, list problem areas.
- Treat yourself to a food regimen of whole, pure, and natural foods.
- Avoid using drugs as much as possible. If you have to use pre-scription drugs, ask your doctor to prescribe those with the least side effects.
- Ease out of destructive, stressful relationships at home and work. Learn to stand up to—or get away from—abusive, criti-

cal people. You need to be around people who really love and respect you.

- Slow down the rate of romantic involvement with any persons until you find out where they are coming from and what they are like. Ask what their family life was like when they were growing up. If they were mistreated or ignored, realize they might need counselling to deal with emotional scars that could cause problems in their relationship with you.
- Find a job in which you can feel good about yourself and those you work with, even if it means less pay.
- If you are married, improve the way you deal with your mate first. Then, begin working on problem areas together. Get help from a marriage counselor if necessary.
- If your friends are not loving people, ask yourself what you are doing with them and why. Someone who doesn't care about you is not your friend. Don't allow yourself to be somebody else's unhealthy "fix" or dumping ground.
- If you have children, spend quality time with them and begin easing them into a healthier diet and healthier snacks. Make sure they know you love them. Ask them about their friends and what they do in school. Be sure you know what's going on in their lives. This applies for both parents if you are married.
- Make your home—especially your bedroom—as beautiful as you can on your budget. Make it into the kind of environment you enjoy, one that reflects your tastes and personality.
- If you realize that you have emotional or moral problems that you can't deal with, get professional help. Try to find a church or synagogue where the people love and care for one another. Keep going until they know you well enough to include you in their activities—this seldom happens instantly (even though it should). It's worth the work to keep at it.
- Make it your goal in life to be a healthy, loving person, not only to lovers or your mate, but to friends and strangers.
- Be careful and be aware of your weaknesses. Don't allow yourself to be taken advantage of.
- Promiscuity is unhealthy—not to mention dangerous these days. Monogamous marriages work best. So don't play around, if only for the sake of your health.

Chapter Three
Love and Sex—
All in the Mind

When we stop and think about it, we find that the body is a servant of the mind, molding to the mind's expression. There was never a smile that didn't start in the mind first. There was never a frown that didn't begin with a thought. We wink in the mind before the eyelid moves; a kiss is a feeling before it is anything else. If we only understood the vast power we hold in the mental realm, all aspects of life would become much simpler, much more harmonious.

We have to recognize that without the love and tenderness that flow from our mental response to our partner there is no "good sex." Physical sex alone is one-dimensional, one-sided; an unabashed exhibition of selfish pleasure-seeking or biological compulsion. Love and sex should not be one partner getting what he or she can from the other person, giving as little as possible in return. Sex should not be a dehumanizing, insensitive act, an insult to the spirit of man.

Instead, sex should be full of sensitivity expressed in the context of a real love relationship, where it will feed not only the spirit of the lovers, but that of the love relationship itself.

THE MIND IS THE NAVIGATOR

One of the foremost reasons why we must take care of what goes into and what comes out of the mind is that the mind is the logical, emotional, ethical, and moral navigator of the body. A good many of our physical problems originate in spiritual, psychic, and mental snarls. If we took care of them at the level of the mind, they would never get to the body.

Doctors now recognize that many physical diseases are psychosomatic in origin and that all diseases have some psychosomatic effects. The word *psychosomatic* comes from the Greek words *psyche* (mind) and *soma* (body). What we accept, what we believe, goes first into the mind before it moves into the flesh. The so-called "sins of the flesh" are all originally from the mind, and this is where we have to straighten things out.

In virtually all cases of sexual system malfunction, sexual dissatisfaction, lovelessness, loneliness, coldness, marital conflict, sex crimes, deviation, glandular imbalance, and any other aspect of human sexuality you can think of, we vastly underestimate the mind's role in the emergence of the problem and the mind's capacity to contribute to the solution of the problem. I should mention here that nutrition—what we eat and drink—strongly influences our mental life. But even the power to choose nutritious food and drink is in the mind, is it not?

There must be a meeting of the minds before there can be a mating of the bodies. People can so easily grow apart when they neglect to "tune in" to each other's needs, desires, and interests. And neglect tends to be contagious. When one partner senses indifference in the other, the initial response may be hurt feelings; the eventual response will be an equal and opposite case of indifference.

Like the body, the mind has certain inherent strengths and weaknesses. Like the body, the mind needs certain foods to function in a healthy way, and when it is fed properly, the inherent weaknesses do not break down or become diseased. Some years ago black people in this country coined the term "soul food." People of all races need "soul food" to have healthy minds, healthy love lives, healthy sex lives.

What is "soul food"? We feed the mind with beauty, truth, color, lovely experiences, perfume, music, delicious tastes, the things we love to touch, graceful movements, poetry, art, learning, satisfying work, a sense of achievement, and love. To a great extent, our ability to appreciate "soul food" for the mind depends on our earliest experiences.

INFLUENCES ON THE MIND

Your mind, as it exists right now, is influenced by three main factors: your genetic inheritance; your childhood home environment; and your education and experience. Sometimes it is difficult to tell whether we have inherited a certain personality trait from our mother or father, or just picked it up from being around them so much. Whether we can actually distinguish between the two doesn't matter. What matters is to realize that these influences have been at work in the mind.

Look back on your parents, your upbringing. Were you loved? In what ways did your parents show love toward you? Toward each other? Were they reluctant to show affection toward you? Toward each other in front of their children?

There is no doubt that the way parents act toward one another and toward their children influences the way the children act when they grow up. Unfortunately, failure to provide a visible example of love is certainly a serious omission and is difficult to overcome. But the curse can be broken. We can all learn to love, no matter what our background.

My father was a rough man, a man with a terrific temper, and a perfectionist. It was hard for us kids to see love coming from a man who was so ready to respond harshly when we did something he disapproved of. We were afraid of him. As a child, I

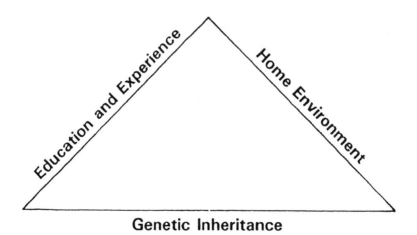

The Triangle of the Mind

stuttered and stammered and, at least to some degree, I believe this was connected to my relationship with my father. Looking back, I believe he loved us, in his own way. But, from a child's innocent perspective, I couldn't tell.

Love starvation is very hard on the mind, especially on the emotions. Of all forms of stress, it may be the cruelest, the most difficult to bear. Without love, a person can become almost inhuman in his or her behavior—if he or she allows it. We don't have to allow it. We can break the "love starvation syndrome" by reaching out to someone else, by touching another life, and by offering love.

Some of us fear expressing love because we are afraid of rejection. Perhaps in the past, parents turned away from the child's offer of or need for love. Or, perhaps we have been spurned too many times by those we loved. If you are one of these, you need to know there is someone who will receive your love. Don't be afraid to seek the right person, for the right person will love you in return. We are all vulnerable when we offer or ask for love. There is no "safe" way to give or receive love. We are all made to love and we must love—for our own good.

Children of divorced parents frequently have problems with relationships when they grow up. When the reason for the divorce involves an alcoholic parent, wife beating, or child abuse, the children's later problems are compounded beyond the consequences of divorce alone. Memories of fear, pain, and frequent distress tend to make children insecure when they grow into adults, fearful of abandonment by their partner, overly jealous, untrusting, and uneasy with intimacy.

There are those who have suffered sexual abuse as children, and they almost always need counselling to help heal the terrifying memory of that time. Many marriages have broken up simply because a wife who had been raped or abused as a child could not tolerate sexual relations with her husband and felt unable to tell him of the incident or get the proper counselling. *Always* seek professional counsel if you have been a victim of sexual violence.

Many of us look for the ideal person to marry. The ideal may be composed of characteristics we liked in our fathers or mothers, together with characteristics opposite to those we disliked, feared, or hated in them. This ideal may include bits and pieces of characters from fairy tales, films, TV, and real-life models such as teachers. The most important thing to know about an ideal image is that once we fall in love with the dream, every real person is going to fall short of it. We can't fall in love with a real person when an image is blocking the view.

What are we seeing as we consider the various obstacles to love that can grow out of childhood? Love isn't easy for everyone, is it? Is it easy for you? If not, you will need to take a good look at whatever is hindering you from expressing love fully in your life, especially toward your mate and your children. Bad memories can be overcome. Personality problems can be overcome. Behavioral problems can be overcome. It is comforting—indeed inspiring—to realize that the solution lies beside every problem in life.

SEX EDUCATION

Another major influence on the development of our attitudes toward love and sex comes from our schools. I'm not sure these programs have been a great success. There are more unwed mothers than ever before, despite most teenagers' being informed about birth control and "the pill." There are more cases of sexually-transmitted diseases than ever before, despite clear teaching in the schools about what they are, how they are passed along, and how to prevent them. The current epidemics of venereal herpes and AIDS are cases in point, and no cure has been found for them yet.

We find that information and knowledge, by itself, is not sufficient to change a young person's sexual behavior. The average American male has his first sexual experience at age 15, the average female at age 16. In one southern California high school, 150 out of the 880 girls in the student body became pregnant in a single year. This is sad. The great majority of teenage marriages are due to unanticipated pregnancy, and many teenage mothers do not get married at all. Teenagers are not noted for their wisdom, responsibility, or ability to handle problems. Therefore, society pays for the mistakes its parents, schools, and teenagers make.

Parents are divided over sex education in the public schools because they disagree over the moral issues involved and because they disagree over the impact they feel sex education may have on their children. Some parents don't object to teen sexual experiences, but only want their children to be protected from unwanted pregnancy and venereal disease. Other parents object to premarital sex on moral grounds and believe that sexually-explicit information encourages sexual experimentation.

Obviously, our children need to learn about human sexuality. They need the kind of learning environment that will encourage them to make wise decisions about their own sexuality and to avoid experiences that have serious adverse consequences. Too many of our young people today are getting hurt by early sexual experiences that rob them of future hope and happiness. They need to be able to cope with their own sexuality much more realistically and effectively than they are now doing.

Teenagers used to get most of their information about sex from one another. More rarely, they were told about sex by their parents. There was much misinformation and inadequate information brought out in this way, but sex problems then were not as widespread or serious as they are now when the schools are teaching the "correct" information. So, we ask, "What are we doing wrong?"

SEXUAL "MALNUTRITION"

I believe most teenagers today—and perhaps their parents, too—have stopped believing in the moral values that should be taught even before sex information is presented. Or perhaps the moral values are not being taught in a meaningful way. Despite these shortcomings, I am wondering if sex should not be taught in the churches, along with moral values that help children learn to exercise self-control. At the same time, we must not teach that sex is "dirty" or "sinful."

As a child, I faced the painful task of sorting through a cruel heap of condemning accusations laid on me in the guise of religious truth. I was told I was conceived in sin, born in sin, was living in sin, and would die in sin. I was told I was no good and that sex was sin. Because of this indoctrination, I can personally attest that to see all sexual functions and feelings as sinful is very confusing and upsetting to children. As a child, I wondered how it could be possible to be morally clean and still fall in love. I wondered how it was possible for someone with a spiritually-pure mind to think of sex, even in marriage. "Do we have to be celibate to be sinless?" I'd ask myself. It took me many years to realize that what I was told was a harsh and distorted misinterpretation of religious values.

Although sex is considered to be triggered by physical desire, desire starts in the mind. And the mind does not deal well with sexual desire unless basic moral and ethical values and the will to obey them are present. Unless moral and ethical values are taught along with "the facts of life," the facts of life for teenagers are going to be increasingly dismal.

We have to get across to our young people that love and sex are more than the fun, recreational activity they are promoted to be by movies, TV, and popular literature. Sex is the body's version of love, an act designed for procreation and joy, one of the highest experiences of man. It is meant to be shared by mature adults who know who they are, and who are capable of taking full responsibility for their action and the consequences of those actions.

Seeking love and sexual fulfillment outside a moral framework is like eating from an empty plate. We may go through the motions, but when it is over, we are just as starved for what we really need as when we began. Many of our teenagers (and many adults as well) do not realize that love and sex are far more than a physical act. Man is body, mind, and spirit—a whole being—and the sexual experience affects the mind and spirit as well as the body. The Good Book refers to sex as the most intimate knowledge we can have of another person. Intimate in what sense? Certainly, it is intimate at the physical level, but I believe it is also intimate at the mental and spiritual levels.

It is clear to me that love and sex are very much in the mind as well as the body. There is a sex center in the brain in the hypothalamus, and it is affected by what we eat; by our circulation; by our blood; and by what we think, sense, and feel. Most of these factors are determined early in our lives by our genes and childhood experiences. We have to take care of our brain centers if we expect our bodies to function properly. We have to feed the brain, exercise it, and allow it to express our individuality through the proper activities.

We feed the mind with beauty, color, lovely music, natural sounds and scenes, delightful odors and perfumes, wonderful thoughts and feelings. We need emotional satisfaction as much or more than we need physical satisfaction. We need to love and be loved; we need true friends; we need fulfilling work, work that offers an outlet for our gifts, talents, and skills. We need to express our emotions and to be around others who express theirs. We need to avoid spiteful people as much as possible. We need to think clearly and deal honestly with all men and women we meet.

We find that what we believe governs much of our thought life, so we must be careful what we believe. My mother used to say, "If you believe a lie, you live a lie." Learn to incorporate the highest moral and ethical values into your life; live by them, think by them. A person who is without guilt or shame because he or she leads a clean life and keeps the mind clean has peace of mind, perhaps the greatest brain food of all.

Chapter Four
What Attracts People to One Another?

I believe there are universal laws that control the way men and women are attracted to one another. This may not sound very romantic at first. I assure you that it is delightfully romantic, as you'll soon see.

There's a whole body of interesting folklore on romantic attraction. Do gentlemen really prefer blondes? Are redheads, in fact, more fun? Do Latins make better lovers? Are the French more sophisticated about matters of the heart than other people? I have to confess I don't know the answers to these questions, and I doubt if anyone else does, either.

One prevailing romantic ideal has been that of a gallant prince riding upon his white steed to sweep his princess off her feet; the two ride off into the sunset to live happily ever after. Women have been looking for their dream princes for as long as I can remember. Men have been searching for their princesses at least since the turn of the century. When we think of romance, we may think of the late movie actress Grace Kelly when she married Prince Ranier of Monaco; or of Britain's "Di" and "Fergie" who became royalty when they married British Princes Charles and Andrew. But real life is not romantic perfection—even for them.

What the "prince" and "princess" ideal boils down to, really, is the hope for an ideal mate, the man or woman of our dreams. Each young man and young woman has a preconceived notion of the ideal mate, the kind of person he or she would like to fall in love with. Where does this mental picture come from, and what influences our choice of a partner?

LEFT BRAIN AND RIGHT BRAIN ACTIVITIES

The two hemispheres of the brain may hold the answer to an important part of our question, "What attracts people to one another?" The left hemisphere of the brain is said to be the rational, thinking, and analytic side of the brain, while the right hemisphere is more concerned with emotion, beauty, music, and feelings. Men are thought to be somewhat dominated by left-brain activity, like solving math problems or working with tools, while it is often speculated that women are dominated by right-brain functions—like socializing or painting.

Men and women are created with many qualities in common, among them strength, intelligence, love, hope, ambition, and appreciation for beauty. But they are also created to complement one another. Each sex has qualities lacking in the other. Allowing for differences among individuals, it is still fair to state a few generalities that are *relatively* true of each sex. Men are harder, stronger, tougher, more aggressive. Women are softer, more giving and sensitive, more compassionate. Men value reason more highly than feelings. Women value feelings more highly than reason.

Perhaps we could compare the two types of behavior to the two poles of a magnet, the left-brain activity (stronger in men) attracting, and attracted to, the right-brain functions (stronger in women). Together, the two form a completely balanced union.

But, beyond this mental attraction, men and women must work to create more permanent bonds.

THE ROLE OF AFFINITIES IN LOVE

To begin, let's say affinities are common interests and compatibilities that attract people to one another to assure a sustained relationship. These affinities may be second only to love in creating the bonds that keep a relationship healthy, enjoyable, and—in the case of marriage—permanent.

I believe that the human body is the physical vehicle used by the immortal soul to develop and grow. The interplay of affinities between two human beings is part of that growth and development. It is extremely important.

Often, love is not enough to sustain a relationship beyond the infatuation stage. We need affinities, shared interests. We become very unhappy when our potentials are unfulfilled, ignored, neglected, or rejected. We must be able to feel comfortable with a person and share experiences so we can learn and grow as we should.

To make a physical comparison, the cells of our bodies have natural affinities to the chemical elements and nutrients they need to accomplish their function and stay healthy. As these nutrients flow through the bloodstream, cells draw them out of the blood by electromagnetic affinity. If the right chemical elements aren't there, the cell cannot be properly nourished, cannot perform its functions properly, and cannot remain healthy. Similarly, a relationship between a man and a woman that does not match or fulfill each of their affinities cannot remain healthy.

Socrates taught "Know Thyself" as the most important law of life. For a relationship to be successful, I believe a couple should make up comprehensive lists of what they like and dislike, including goals, hopes, ambitions, attitudes, and possibly every other aspect of life they consider important. The lists of two persons should have at least a 70 percent correlation before they marry, no matter how much they love one another. Love, alone, is not enough to make a healthy marriage.

Affinities may include a shared fondness for foods, sports, hobbies, books, TV programs, pets, art, climate, houses, recreation, work, skills, music, cars, lifestyle, habits, religion, and many other things. It isn't enough for both to be attracted to music. If one partner likes hard rock and the other likes classical, they will clash. It isn't enough for both to be attracted to religion. If one person is Moslem and the other is Christian, they will disagree.

Complementary affinities are different from mutual interests. A complementary affinity is a quality that one person must have to get along with a person who has a different, sometimes nearly opposite, quality or affinity. For example, a critical husband needs a tolerant wife. A bashful person needs a more confident mate to draw him or her out. A careless, sloppy person needs a tolerant, orderly person as a mate. Affinities such as approval and enjoyment are priceless to those who need to feel the support of their mates on what they do. For example, a body builder probably needs a mate who really likes body builders. The same is true of a race car driver, a circus performer, or a lawyer.

Mates who are "right" for us have the ability to "quicken" us, to motivate and encourage us to do better at almost anything we do. Children are nearly always more excited, enthusiastic, and motivated about their actions when an adult is watching and appreciating them.

We still carry some of this childlike trait into adulthood. We all enjoy having people pay attention to us and like what we are doing. We also recognize that it takes a certain kind of partner to bring the best out of us. Think of how unhappy a marriage would be where the wife needed a lot of encouragement and praise but the husband never gave it. Let's remember, however, that we need to work at fulfilling each other's lives—not just our own.

I want to add that very few affinities are permanently fixed, unvarying qualities. Even music lovers can appreciate silence at times, and the most critical persons give praise. A bashful person may make a bold statement, and a confident man can be crushed by a critical remark. If affinities are viewed as tendencies rather than permanent characteristics, they are still affinities. We want them. We enjoy them. We need and seek them out in a person to whom we are attracted.

The purpose of love is to find completion in companionship at the physical, mental, and spiritual levels. Love is not, in itself, sexual. But it cannot be separated from sexuality because both are expressed through the same body and the same mind.

When I say love is "discriminating," I mean it is selective in its object, as compared with sex. The soul hungers for wholeness, and it looks for the right person to fulfill the love relationship. Love works through both the rational, analytical left brain, and the emotional, intuitive right brain, looking for those elements in another person that bring fulfillment. Remember, fulfillment is a two-way process—we can't really be fulfilled unless we also fulfill what needs to be completed in the other person.

If love is repressed and sexual expression is emphasized, life is limited to a very shallow, superficial affair. The sex drive provides the power for love to be expressed in passion. By itself, love lacks force; by itself, sex lacks direction. Love provides the direction for sex to be creative and fulfilling. The sex drive alone responds only to the body, but love responds to the whole person.

OUR SECRET ATTRACTIONS

If we acknowledge that allergies can be triggered by substances so small we don't see, hear, feel, smell, or taste them, surely we can recognize that we may be attracted to or repelled from a person by factors that we don't consciously recognize. These are what we call subliminal factors.

As we have pointed out earlier, moths and other insects, and most animals, exude sexual chemicals (called pheromones) that can attract a mate from long distances. In recent years perfume and cologne manufacturers, in the process of experiments to discover chemicals that will attract one human to another, have found that men and women already possess subtle, natural odors that attract the opposite sex. Is it possible that we recognize a compatible mate on the basis of subliminal cues like pheromones?

Similarly, most of us have favorite colors and respond favorably to those who wear clothing of colors we like. In most cases we may not be aware of the reason why we are attracted to certain people, only that we are aroused.

While moths and other creatures can attract a mate from miles away, human senses tend to become more acute when we are in the immediate vicinity of a potential mate. In fact, physical closeness is the first and probably most necessary ingredient for attraction. Usually, the more you are near someone, the more you are attracted to that person. Certainly the smells, sounds, and sight of another person can hold a powerful attraction for us; can even affect us subliminally and can be crucial in our selection of a mate. But of all the senses, that of touch is the most intimate.

I've seen scientific photographs of a young man's and young women'a fingertips before and during a kiss. While they were kissing, bright energy flares developed around their fingertips that were not present before they kissed. I am sure that the touch for someone who really cares for another is sensed differently than the touch of one who doesn't care; and we respond differently in each case.

How another person touches us is as important as the touch itself. Is the touch sensitive and relaxed, or tense, and restrained? Our feelings toward someone we know may predispose us to feel pleasure or repulsion at his or her touch. If the touch is from someone we don't know well, usually that touch tells us something about the person. We experience certain feelings during and after the touch that determine whether we are attracted or not.

However, we should be careful about touching. Some people don't like to be touched, especially by strangers, and no matter what your intentions are, your touch will not be appreciated.

A WORD TO THE WISE ABOUT ATTRACTION

It should be obvious by now that the practical function of sexual attractiveness is to draw those of the opposite sex into your vicinity so you can find out more about them and give useful feedback about yourself. Then you can tell if the relationship is worth putting more energy into. If all you are interested in is sex, the relationship will seldom develop into more than a superficial interaction with a high eventual probability of disappointment, frustration, and pain.

Warning: When dates or parties involve high levels of alcohol consumption or drug use, your personality and that of your companion will be altered, masked (or both) by the effects of chemicals on your brain. Typically, this results in projecting your imagined expectations on your date, making him or her *seem* more attractive than he or she really is. Romantic or sexual feelings under those circumstances can be terribly misleading. Therefore, if you meet someone you think you like at a party where drugs or alcohol are freely used, arrange to see that person later when there is no chemical alteration or masking of personality. Personally, I am opposed to excess drinking and drug use because of their effects on health, behavior, the mind, and relationships.

Learn to be wise about attractiveness—your own and that of the opposite sex. You'll be much happier in the long run if you do. Following are some tips on being genuinely attractive.

- Let your joy and enthusiasm about the little things in life show in your smiles and laughter.
- Show appreciation for everything you enjoy, and you'll be appreciated.
- Let your love for others be the "no strings attached" kind.
- Be quick to praise, slow to criticize. If you don't agree with someone, you can remain silent. But be a good listener.
- Know your best colors and best scent (perfume, cologne, etc.). You'll feel more like enjoying yourself when you like how you look and smell.
- Consciously decide to be a happy person.
- Decorate your home to reflect your taste, with touches that will please others.
- Be yourself—but be the best that's in you, to attract the best in others.
- Believe you are worth loving.

Chapter Five
Words—Loving or Unloving Vibrations

Actress Marlene Dietrich once said, "Tenderness is greater proof of love than the most passionate of vows." Most of us are familiar with the old adage, "Action speaks louder than words." Yet what we say as well as what we do determines the quality of our relationships and the success or failure of our marriages.

In any language, the words "I love you" are understood as one of the greatest and deepest expressions of affection possible. When these words come from the heart, they carry a loving vibration more powerful than any other statement a person can make. By contrast, the words "I don't love you anymore," can cut a person to the quick, stabbing like an icy knife into a tender, unsuspecting heart. We might say that "I love you" is a creative vibration. Conversely, we could say that "I don't love you anymore" is a destructive vibration. At least that's how these declarations are perceived by the listener.

Words can create pictures in the imagination, stimulate the sensations of taste, smell, touch, and hearing so that what we are reading or hearing becomes almost real to us. Words can stir passions to a raging fire; and words can calm an emotional storm. Words can record the past, express the present, and reach out for the future. Words have both started wars and stopped them. Words have a tremendous impact on our daily lives, our relationships, and our marriages. Communication between lovers—or the lack of it—is perhaps the key ingredient in developing complete and enduring relationships.

WORDS ARE SEEDS THAT GROW

Just as food nourishes the body as it passes through, words nourish the soul and spirit. Truth nourishes the higher faculties. Lies damage them. That's why truth, honesty, and integrity are so important to a relationship. A person must first understand his or her true self, then communicate that truth to the world. When we tell a lie or believe a lie, part of our life becomes a lie. We lose the true sense of our own identity and our own destiny. And without a true sense of our own identity, there is no chance of forming a harmonious relationship with another person's mind and spirit.

When we speak loving thoughts to others, we become loving people. When we speak hateful thoughts to others—or even *think* hateful thoughts—we become hateful people. Loving words and thoughts are health-building as well as character-building. Hateful words and thoughts are destructive to the health and to the character. Words are seeds that have tremendous potential to grow and affect the minds and spirits of our friends and mates, as well as our own health.

Scientists have researched the connection between our minds and our health, and they have discovered that there are diseases and disturbances that can be triggered by what goes on in our minds. Ulcers, colitis, arthritis, heart disease, and cancer can be triggered, or aggravated, by negative attitudes, thoughts, and feelings. We find that our words reveal what goes on in our minds. I consider this discovery one of the greatest discoveries of our time because if our minds can create conditions destructive to our bodies and lives, they can also create and support good health, beneficial lifestyles, and happy, healthy, relationships.

OUR WORDS SHOULD LIFT OTHERS

Everyone has at least a few positive characteristics and lifestyle qualities. If we relate to others on the basis of their best qualities—instead of criticizing or trying to correct their worst qualities—their level of thinking about themselves is elevated. Thus, their worst qualities are gradually changed for the better. Change starts in the mind first before it is expressed in behavior or conversation.

In your relationships with others, you will communicate more effectively if you focus on their positive traits. Remember, though, you can help another person change only if you make it

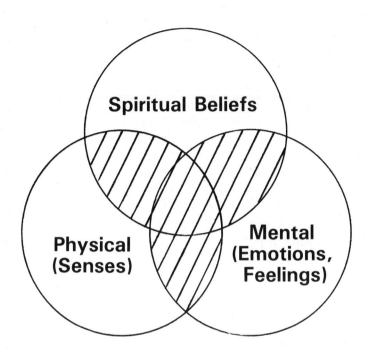

Three Related Spheres. Loving vibrations (overlapping area) can speak to the physical, mental, and spiritual union of love. Loving vibrations are positive, complimentary, and honest. Our ultimate goal would be to have all three areas completely overlap.

possible for them to change themselves. We can't really change people ourselves.

As you know, most advice is useless. Criticism may make a person feel bad or respond with anger, but it won't make the person change. In fact, changing the other person isn't really a worthwhile goal. Life is a process in which each of us tries to grow into our highest potential as a human being. Perhaps the only true way to grow is by helping others become the best they can be.

By strengthening the best qualities in ourselves and others, negative qualities diminish and positive qualities grow. When a person feels good about himself or herself, being angry, jealous, anxious, worried, depressed, or frightened becomes very difficult.

COMMUNICATION

The experts say that men tend to talk more in terms of facts, while women talk more in terms of feelings. One survey of married couples showed that the great majority of women wished their husbands would talk more about their feelings. This is especially evident in times of disagreements. Men tend to develop logical reasons to support their side of the argument. Women talk about their feelings. If men talked about how they felt about their reasons, and if women talked about the reasons for their feelings, disagreements would be resolved much more often.

Facts and feelings are both important, but psychologists have found that feelings are more effective in getting a person to do something—or to stop doing something.

When a person's actions upset you, it doesn't do much good to accuse or give reasons not to act that way. The best way to respond is, "When you do such-and-such, I feel so-and-so." For example, "When you forget to phone me, I feel very hurt." Or, "When you track mud on the rug, I really feel angry." It doesn't work as well to say, "You make me angry when you track mud on the rug," because the accusation "You make" is a *blaming statement*. People don't respond well to blaming statements.

Blaming statements are ineffective in changing behavior for at least two reasons. First, "You make me feel such-and-such" stirs up a resentment reaction. Second, blaming statements focus on the person rather than the event that triggered your emotional response. This generates a negative feeling—usually anger in the one you're talking to. What you're suggesting with blaming statements is that the other person is responsible for your feelings. This simply isn't true.

We're all responsible for our own feelings. It's nice to know that *feeling statements* not only help people change bad habits but also strongly encourage good habits. "When you take me out to dinner, I feel so appreciative. I just love it." This is the way to build up a happy relationship. It is especially effective if you follow your feeling statement with action—such as a kiss or a hug.

Feeling statements are also effective in helping people change their emotional patterns, but you have to be careful. For example, it may be appropriate to say, "When you get angry like that, I feel frightened," unless the goal of the person in displaying anger is actually to frighten you. In this case, you must change directions.

When a person is showing signs of strong emotion, especially if you're not sure what the cause is, often your best tactic is to show him you are aware of his emotion. You start by saying, ''You're really angry.'' Then stop and give the person a chance to respond. Your goal is to get him to talk about it, to release the pressure of the feeling in a safe way. If he doesn't respond to your recognition statement after the opportunity is presented, say, ''What happened?'' or ''Tell me about it.'' Then be a good listener.

Whether the emotion is anger, fear, hurt, resentment, or other such feelings, a big hug can make a powerful change. In any case, when the other person begins talking, be a good listener. Men, especially, need to resist breaking in with advice on what to do—whether they're listening to a woman or another man. Don't offer advice unless and until it is asked for. When people are emotionally aroused, they need to express that emotion much more than they need advice about the situation that caused the emotion.

Do not encourage or insist that another person suppress or ignore his emotions. This is emotionally and physically unhealthy. It could also bring a backlash onto you, perhaps at a later time. Don' ever reject or deny another person's feelings. Feelings are real, and even if you are uncomfortable with the particular feeling the other person is expressing, don't pretend the feeling isn't there. Feelings are natural responses to real-life situations.

Men are guilty of suppressing feelings more often than women and are often uncomfortable in the presence of someone who is expressing a strong emotion, such as grief, sadness, shame, or frustration. Fathers sometimes try to give their children orders about their emotions. ''Stop crying,'' they say. Or, ''Wipe that smile off your face'' or ''I'll do it for you.'' Or, ''Shut up or you'll get a good spanking.'' This is very unhealthy for the child and for the child-parent relationship. It's also a poor idea to try to bribe an emotion away from someone. ''If you stop crying, I'll take you to a movie.''

If you notice that someone has been expressing an emotion for what may be too long, you may want to distract him or her in some way. Try taking a walk together, playing a game, or having a snack. There is such a thing as overemotionalism. It is not healthy. Try to help the person get to a better place with his or her feelings.

LOVING OR UNLOVING WORDS

Being in love is, by its very nature, a highly vulnerable and very sensitive time. The words of a loved one have an impact that is beyond understanding. A small compliment may bring joy, while the slightest criticism may result in great offense and, possibly, a temporary break in the relationship. Everything that is said flows into the memory. Whether it is consciously remembered later, or not, does not matter. It is stored in the memory and will—consciously or unconsciously—affect the relationship in later times.

At the same time, it is of the utmost importance for a love relationship to begin with honesty and sincerity. You must be yourself so the other person can relate to the "real" you. I'm not saying you shouldn't be on your best behavior; be sympathetic and very courteous toward the one you love. But if you put on such a false front that the other person is falling in love with that false front and not the real you, you will face great difficulty later on.

Very few people are expert communicators or skilled conversationalists when they are young, yet you should be aware of the importance of your words. Much of your conversation should be spent finding out about the other person, not in boasting about what a great person you are. If you can't impress the one you love by being yourself, and you resort to exaggerations, or talk about the wealth of your family of the famous people you know, you are in for deep trouble later on. You are inviting your lover to fall in love with an image, a reputation, and not a person. Images have a way of tarnishing, and reputations fall when flaws in the person appear later—and everyone has flaws. You don't have to let yourself fall in love with an image, and you don't have to present yourself as a bigger-than-life person to the one you love. Guard against it by making sure the one you love knows the real you. You'll be glad you did later on.

I do not propose that you should present your loved one with a list of your bad habits and personal flaws. But don't try to hide anything in your life that might create a sense of shock, disappointment, or surprise later on when the one you love finds out. Similarly, don't be surprised to find out that the man or woman you love has flaws. Be glad you're not in love with a "perfect" person, because you would never be able to live with one. You'd feel too self-conscious and too "imperfect" by comparison to be comfortable in the relationship.

Words have a tendency to create an emotional climate which either nourishes or diminishes a relationship. Words come from an emotional and attitudinal context when you say them, and they have an emotional impact on the one you are talking to. In a very important sense, words are loving or unloving vibrations, making a direct impact on the mind and spirit of the person to whom you are speaking. In that mind, love is expressed toward you, and your words either build that love up or tear it down. You end up being the winner or loser, simply by the way you treat the other person.

Unconditional love—that is, love with no strings attached—is the ideal. Ideally, we should love whether we're loved in return or not. But there is no relationship unless you are loved in return. Unloving words can kill a relationship suddenly or gradually. Your unloving words directly affect *you*—through the response you elicit from the other person. Be loving—and be careful.

Chapter Six
Awakening the Love Consciousness

Each of us has a number of gifts, talents, and faculties that we are born with, and these are part of our genetic inheritance. They remain latent in our brain structure until they are awakened and developed at the proper time and in the proper circumstances of our lives. These gifts, talents, and faculties may include music, mathematics, art, poetry, business, hospitality, leadership, and many other things—not the least of which is love.

Experience—not only mine but that of many others as well—has shown that these inherent potentials may require awakening and nurturing before they flower into fullness of expression. For example, many people with an exceptional gift for music have never had that gift fully awakened or developed because they were too busy making a living, or because they emphasized other gifts, talents, and faculties and never got around to realizing their musical potential.

We have to understand that our gifts, talents, and various faculties are expressed most fully when we have developed the channels through which they work. The artist must have a sharp eye for color and proportion. The musician should have an ear tuned for music. The gymnast should have a well-developed sense of timing, coordination, and finely tuned muscle development.

When we realize that love involves the emotions, and that we live on what we give forth, we must realize we must also have a balanced glandular system and good nerves to help us experience awakening of the love consciousness. This is why we have to understand the role of nutrition, exercise, and the other elements of a healthy lifestyle. To love, as to express any other gift, we need to be in top shape. We need a healthy body, a clear mind, and a positive spirit to be the best we can be.

Some gifts require awakening by another person or persons. For instance, a leader can't become a leader until he or she has developed a following. One with a gift for mathematics requires a teacher to guide the student through the inherent technicalities. Similarly, the gift of love requires an object, a "target," another person, to help it to fully awaken.

LOVE IS A RAINBOW

There are many expressions of love in each person's life. Children may love their parents, their toys, and their pets. We may say we love to go window shopping, hiking, or sight-seeing. We may love art, poetry, or nature. These are kinds of love in which we invest or involve ourselves with some object or process, and we feel pleasure as a consequence. It isn't that these things are only forms of selfishness, because we often learn to respond to what we love, to care for something outside ourselves, to give time and effort toward taking care of the things we love. For example, a child with a pet learns to play with it, feed it, pet it. The child learns to respond to a pet's needs and to do things that make the pet happy.

A baby first learns love from its mother. The feeding, the warmth of the mother's body, the comforting sound of her voice are each important aspects of awakening the love consciousness. More importantly, a baby can sense when it is loved. I believe there is a fine, high-frequency electromagnetic field generated by love, and babies intuitively recognize and respond to that "love field." Similarly, babies seem to sense anger, fear, jealousy, kindness, and other feelings in adults. They respond uniquely to each of these vibrations, fussing and crying at the negative vibrations, cooing and smiling at the positive vibrations.

When a newborn baby is deprived of motherly love by being cared for in an institution such as a hospital, for example, it is deprived of this very important "awakening" process. I'm not saying that people in institutions don't love the babies they take care of. I'm pointing out that many people are involved, and even though they love the babies, workers are changed every eight-hour shift. Babies never develop that sense of "connection" or "intimacy" with one person that the experience with a mother fosters.

Children both see and sense the love their parents have for each other. They watch to see how mothers and fathers express their love—the touching of hands; the hugs, kisses, warm looks at each other; the tones of voice. Children sense when one or both parents stop loving the other, or when they are angry or jealous. Children become anxious and uneasy when they sense an absence of love or the presence of negative emotions between parents.

Similarly, children learn to love their brothers, sisters, aunts, uncles, cousins, and grandparents—and they experience being loved by them. This, too, is part of the awakening of the love consciousness.

Awareness of our love consciousness helps us to build on our initial experiences of love. Most of us remember the heart pangs, the rush of feeling that accompanied our first adolescent love. Whether we developed our first "boyfriend-girlfriend" relationship then, or kept our feelings secret, doesn't matter. The lesson is the same. Most of us learn this lesson—what a powerful thing love is—while still in our teens.

FORMATION OF THE LOVE CONSCIOUSNESS

We find that many adults of all ages have difficulty with love and the expression of love in their sex life. Many times this can be traced to childhood experiences.

If any of the childhood family experiences that first serve to awaken the child's love consciousness are absent or distorted, the child's ability to love and respond to love may be repressed, delayed, or deviated from normal. It can never be destroyed, but it can be injured or altered, and this shows up in the adult later on.

The most obvious injuries and wounds to a child's love consciousness come from child abuse (either physical or tongue-lashing), incest, neglect (by one or both parents), and from divorce or separation of the parents. If a child observes physical or verbal abuse between parents—either directly or peripherally, such as by listening from another room—the effect on the child's mind can be devastating. The effects of these types of traumatic experiences can seldom be worked out fully without professional counselling. This is because a powerful memory of pain, betrayal, fear, and mistrust is imbedded in the mind of the child who has witnessed such abuse. Often such childhood memories are stored in the subconscious mind, where they may be forgotten. However, these memories nevertheless remain active and very alive, functioning as a "filter" for all subsequent relationships.

A child's mind is like a very delicate computer. The computer is uniquely designed so each child can have a beautiful, full, and satisfying life, given his particular genetic inheritance. But harsh words, events, and experiences not only go into the memory of that computer, they may also alter its programming. The alteration may not appear for many years after the original experience, or it may make its appearance right away. In any event, when traumatic experiences are imbedded in a child's mind, the child may become unable to respond normally to normal experiences.

Take the story of Evelyn, for example. Evelyn, a child of nine, was raped in a park restroom during a family picnic. The rapist was not found and Evelyn's mother told her to forget it. Evelyn buried this horrible experience in her child's mind and grew up to be a beautiful young woman. She fell in love and seemed to behave normally over the year-and-a-half of the courtship period, responding very affectionately to her fiancé. When they were married, however, their wedding night was disaster. The old "rape" memory destroyed her ability to respond lovingly to her husband. Sex was a nightmare for her. She and her husband were divorced six months later, after trying unsuccessfully to solve the problem on their own.

After two years of psychiatric counselling, Evelyn remarried. This time the marriage was successful.

True, Evelyn's experience at that family picnic was a tragedy. But it does not require a tragedy to influence a child's ability to love. Everyday experiences give children subtle messages, as well. Female children are very affectionate toward their fathers and very observant about how their mothers respond to their fathers. Similarly, male children are very affectionate toward their mothers and very observant about how their fathers act toward their mothers. Notice that the child is not only acting out a loving relationship with a parent of the opposite sex; he or she is watching how the other parent acts. Children learn firsthand about love by how a parent responds to them. They learn secondhand by watching how the parents respond to each other.

LOVE AWAKENS LOVE

At the beginning of this chapter, I suggest that children first learn to love by being loved by their mothers. If an adult does not yet know how to move in the realm of love or has forgotten how, he or she may need a refresher course in accepting love from another person before his or her "love consciousness" can be stimulated or reawakened. You can help reawaken another's love.

We have to reach inside for feelings. We have to reach outside and offer love. We are on this planet to help others to change and become involved in their own lives. If a person has stopped loving, he or she will not move very far in any other area of life until that love is reawakened. Ask yourself then, what needs to happen for this person to experience satisfaction, pleasure, good feelings. You will have to find out how this person can be touched to reawaken their love.

Regardless of life's tragedies, we must not allow the experiences of our past to shape our future beyond our power to choose. A Greek philosopher put it this way: "We never step into the same river twice." Life is change. Life flows on like a river. Each day is a new day. We must recognize that we have the opportunity to start an entirely new life—beginning today. But first, we must move. When something does not move, it is dead. When it dies, we must bury it and go on.

Before we can awaken the love consciousness in another person, we have to first understand and love ourselves. Do you love yourself? We hear a good deal of talk these days about the problems of low self-esteem or, put another way, low self-love. Lack of self-confidence and poor self-image sometimes result because we have been around critical, backbiting people. Sometimes we get down because we took on a task or a job that wasn't right for us, and we failed. Sometimes we may have moved with the wrong crowd and felt inferior simply because we weren't like the others. Or our parents may have rejected us.

None of these events is sufficient to prove that anyone is unworthy. Maybe you need to change your friends. We all need to be around people who appreciate us. Maybe you need to change your job. We all need to work at a job or profession that allows our gifts and talents to be successfully expressed. We all need praise, affirmation, and reassurance so we can feel good about ourselves.

Not everyone is up all the time. When you are down, it is good to be around people who love you, people who will lift you up. If you love someone who is down, then you have an opportunity to lift that person by your actions.

Ironically, there is no better way of breaking out of a feeling of low self-esteem than by helping other people. When we help others, we tend to love ourselves more easily because we sense that inherent value we were born with. We were born to help and serve others.

When we love, the love consciousness is awakened in others. When we sense that love, we are lifted up. When we are lifted up, lifted out of the pit of depression and self-doubt, we begin to love ourselves because we sense our inherent worth. It is then that we can enter into joy, the fullest expression of love's response to life. This is the point where the body, mind, and spirit attain true harmony.

Chapter Seven
Keeping the Body Healthy and Attractive

Our looks reflect the sum total of who we are and how we live, and the best we can do in life is to make the best of what nature has given us, without excuse, apology, or pretense. If we try to live otherwise, we find ourselves acting on a stage with other actors and actresses—great pretenders without real friends, without real lovers, without real relationships.

Most men and women are not as handsome or beautiful as movie stars. Some feel they are too tall and some feel they are too short. Some believe their noses or ears are too big. Any man or woman at certain times feels unattractive. We can all feel "ugly"—to ourselves or others—when we feel uncomfortable, self-conscious, or embarrassed.

THE EYE OF THE BEHOLDER

While we realize that there is such a thing as "natural beauty," which is beyond all standards of culture and history in some sense, there are also "relative" standards of beauty. We all know about fads, styles, and adornments that are "in" one season and "out" the next. This includes cosmetics, hair styles, clothing, and even body weight and size. These standards may vary from country to country, year to year, or even among different age groups in the same country and year. For example, full figures are considered the ideal in some historical periods, but slender figures are valued now—at least in Western countries. Not too many decades ago in China, foot-binding was a very painful custom for young girls, to make them more "attractive." Traditionally, some African tribes enlarge the lips of women by painful forms of stretching, to make them "more beautiful." Tattoos and scarification may have been used as the first "cosmetics" among both sexes and are still popular today in some cultures.

Similarly, in Asia, small nose are considered beautiful (or handsome) while in other cultures, large noses are much preferred. Even within the same cultures standards differ. Here in America, for example, some men prefer buxom women; others prefer the slender, chic type. Some American women prefer muscular men; others prefer slender, more intellectual-looking men.

The point is that cultural standards change—and we may choose to follow or ignore them—because the cultivation of natural beauty is not dependent upon fads.

In order to get along harmoniously, whether at the level of dating, courtship, or marriage, men and women have to get past physical looks and into the more important qualities that make up human relationships, such as kindness, friendship, and areas of mutual interests. There is such a thing as a beautiful personality. There can be beauty in the way a person thinks. An attitude or smile can be beautiful. Love is certainly beautiful, and all of life is beautiful when we are in love. In addition, I believe a person is truly beautiful when he or she is healthy. Any disease or illness affects all parts of the body, sometimes for many years before the symptoms are manifested. If the body and mind are not healthy, then a person cannot feel or be truly attractive. Good health brings a glow to the skin, a ring to the voice, a twinkle to the eye, and a spring to the step that no beauty school can teach.

THE BODY BEAUTIFUL

I don't believe there is anything more beautiful and wonderful than the human body. This is not only my opinion, but that of philosophers, poets, artists, doctors, and countless men and women of all cultures from the beginning of history. Sculptors during the "golden age" of Greece immortalized the human body—both male and female—by creating masterpieces in sculpture that are still considered among the highest forms of art of all time. In our time, TV and magazine ads celebrate the sexuality and beauty of the human body, demonstrating an appeal which is timeless and universal—despite over-commercialization and sometimes tasteless exploitation.

Beauty, whether in nature or art, is always the final outcome of less visible processes. Similarly, the beauty of the human form and personality is vitally dependent on the well-being of our internal organs, and on processes such as blood and lymph circulation, good nerve conduction, brain function, and digestion.

The skin we "love to touch" also happens to be the largest organ in the body, an eliminative organ, like the lungs, kidneys, and bowel. Few people realize that proper bowel habits and good circulation are necessary to keep the skin clean, soft, pliable, free of blemishes, and attractive in appearance. Constipation and underactive elimination are the primary causes of many skin problems because, when bowel function is slowed down, elimination of wastes through the skin is increased.

Vibrant health and beauty are closely related to balanced glandular function. Our endocrine gland system—the pituitary, thyroid, parathyroids, adrenals, and gonad—are essential to what many call "sex appeal." The thyroid gland, for example, by regulating the metabolism, determines the energy level. Energy is life. The most beautiful body in the world is nothing without the energy to let the personality shine through.

We can consider the body as a community of individual organs, glands, and tissues, each a vital part of the whole. When a single organ is not working, the whole body suffers. The brain is especially important, acting as "mayor" to the community of body parts. When all members of the community are working properly and in harmony, life is beautiful. If any is underactive or diseased, the vitality of life is diminished and the expression of beauty is diminished. It is important to take care of the whole body because beauty comes from the inside out.

The Chinese say, "Man is a miracle." In a twenty-four-hour period, the following miraculous events take place in the average person's life:

- You use at least seven million brain cells.
- Your heart beats about 103,689 times.
- You breathe 23,040 times, inhaling and exhaling 438 cubic feet of air.
- Your blood circulates 1,450 times through thousands of miles of arteries, veins, and capillaries.
- You move 750 muscles.
- You eat 3.25 pounds of food and drink 2.9 quarts of liquid.

If all these and thousands of other "miracles" function properly, with each each cell, tissue, and organ performing at its optimum, we are truly beautiful, and our bodies and sexual life are in harmony.

CAN SEX LIFT THE HEALTH LEVEL?

Researchers have long been aware that married people live longer than single or divorced people. A report issued by the American Medical Association reveals that single and divorced men have nearly twice the death rate of married men. A study from Great Britain disclosed that single, widowed, or divorced people are hospitalized more often than married people. That study also revealed that psychiatric and nursing home residents are most often single people.

During the early years of my practice, I noticed that of all my patients, the healthiest and most vital were married couples with active sex lives. I wondered if these people were so sexually active because they were healthy. Or could it be they were healthy because they were so sexually active?

Whatever the catalyst, I concluded that there are many positive correlations between love, sex, and health. For example, I found that an active sex life can help some people cure arthritis; in others, it helps alleviate the pain. Surveys have shown that men and women in love have fewer colds and bouts of flu. Further, those who are sexually active seem to have a higher red blood cell count and better blood circulation. Discoveries like these led me to suspect that hormone changes due to sexual activity were causing these benefits. Certainly, an active sex life seems to help preserve youthfulness.

The reason for this is that sex is both stimulating and rejuvenating to the glandular system. When we make love, the pituitary gland, the thyroid gland, the adrenal glands, the prostate gland and testes in men, and the ovaries in women are thoroughly exercised. The net result is that people in love look and feel better about themselves. They are more self-confident, more assertive. They stand taller, sit straighter, and walk faster. It is also possible that activation of the sex center in the hypothalamus of the brain has health effects on other brain centers. Every cell in the body gets this message and is strengthened by it.

Another way that an active sex life may help prevent disease and illnesses is by strengthening our immune systems. (I should add that the positive effects of being in love—without sex—will probably have the same positive result.)

Various cells of the immune system can destroy tumor and cancer cells, bacteria, viruses, and foreign substances in the blood. The cells of the immune system are the body's main soldiers of defense against outside invaders; without these cells, the body is vulnerable to almost any illness or disease. The critical role played by the immune system has been emphasized dramatically in recent years with the advent of AIDS (which, as most of us know, stands for Acquired Immune Deficiency Syndrome). AIDS is a deadly disease because it destroys the body's immune system, allowing other diseases—such as pneumonia and cancer—to invade and kill with impunity. It is ironic that one of the primary ways the AIDS virus (HIV) is spread is through sexual contact. Thus sexual activity can be the destruction of the immune system (as with the case of AIDS) or can, if it is wholesome, loving sex, nourish and support the immune system.

Scientists have compared the nerve endings of happy, loving, and sexually-fulfilled people with unhappy and sexually-unfulfilled people. Apparently, large numbers of immune-system cells were gathered near the nerve endings in the "happy" people. A similar microscopic exam of "unhappy" and depressed persons showed no such gathering of immune-system cells. Scientists theorize that the nerve endings in the "happy" group were releasing *neurotransmitters*. These are chemicals, like *adrenalin* and *acetylcholine*, that facilitate the transmission of nerve messages. According to their findings, these scientists concluded that these neurotransmitters could attract, feed, and strengthen the various immune-system cells.

We have discussed the positive effects sex has on systemic health. But what about the physiology of sex itself? During sex, the heart beats twice as fast, pumping blood to the pelvis, breasts, nipples, and surface of the skin, helping get rid of toxins and bringing in nutrients. We also breathe twice as fast, bringing in more oxygen. Muscles are tensed and relaxed, alternatively. Of course, not much good is realized by those who rush through lovemaking in ten minutes or less. But for those who spend a leisurely hour or two, the benefits can be considerable.

WATCH YOUR WEIGHT

Of course, love and sex alone do not determine whether or not a person is happy. We need proper diet, fresh air, some sunshine (but remember too much sun ages the skin and can cause skin cancer), exercise, and enough rest. Many of us are now aware that we have to stay away from drugs like nicotine and alcohol that act as chemical depressants. But perhaps the Number One health and beauty concern in the United Sates today, though, is weight control.

Sometimes I wonder whether it is worse to be overweight or to be worried about being overweight. Over 40 percent of Americans are overweight (most of them women), and most are not happy about it. There are several dangers to being overweight. Possibly the greatest danger is trying to reduce too quickly.

I believe that fad diets for "crash" weight loss can take years off a healthy person's life by creating chemical imbalances in the body that adversely affect the heart, liver, glandular system, and brain. Fad diets are usually followed by rapid weight return.

The secret to healthy, permanent weight loss is simple. First, exercise regularly every day, for at least thirty minutes. Second, take weight off slowly, no more than a pound or two per week to allow the body and brain to adjust. Third, diet by using a balanced food regimen and taking smaller portions—or by leaving one-third of your usual helpings on the plate. This way you can stay healthy as you reduce. Fourth, get a friend to exercise and diet with you. Encourage one another to keep motivation high. You can do it.

FOR WOMEN ONLY

If you are one of the millions of women who use cosmetics often, have you ever thought about why you use them?

I do not object in principle to adornment of the skin with the application of various powders, creams, cleansers, color, and highlights. But—in practice—I feel it is dangerous to a person's health to put chemical substances on the skin. We are all exposed to too many dangerous chemicals every day already. I don't believe it is good for anyone's health to put chemical substances on the skin when there are safe alternative methods of enhancing natural beauty. Good health is the most wonderful "cosmetic" a woman can have.

I feel that many times cosmetics are used to cover up the consequences of a poor diet, an unhealthy lifestyle, or an existing health problem that makes the skin and face sallow, rough, dry, broken out, or unattractive in some way. Perhaps the best advice I can give you is just this: learn to accept your body and face and their limitations. Cosmetics cannot hide the "real you" for long, and you must love yourself—with your abilities, talents, and natural beauty—before others will. Once you develop self-confidence in the natural, healthy you, then you will find that cosmetics mean less and less in your life.

Many cosmetics contain substances that bacteria thrive on, and when you use bacteria-loaded cosmetics you can bring on unwanted problems. That's a good reason never to borrow or use anyone else's makeup. If you must use cosmetics, experts say, don't keep creams, oily lotions, or liquid makeup base more than six months. If the consistency of a cream changes (or lumps appear in it), or if an oil-based product begins to smell bad, throw it out. Never use saliva to moisten cake mascara or eye liner, and don't save old mascaras. Instead, buy small mascaras and use them up more quickly. Bacteria are a major problem in mascara and can cause infections in or around the eyes.

Women should sterilize cosmetic brushes by soaking and cleaning them in alcohol. Rinse them with water and wipe dry before using. To reduce bacterial buildup, store cosmetics away from heat and light, in a cool place. Keep lids tight. Wash your hands and face with soap before using cosmetics.

According to California dermatologists, many so-called skin cleansers actually increase skin problems in those who use them, as compared to those who don't. You should avoid skin lotions and cleansers that contain fragrances because they tend to dry out the skin.

I am told that natural cosmetics are coming into vogue, and it is possible that natural cosmetics will be the beauty trend of the future. Meanwhile, there are certain things that will help keep you looking young without risk to your health or complexion.

To keep your face young and beautiful, follow these five simple steps.

1. Avoid prolonged exposure to direct sun and wind.
2. Drink at least six glasses of water each day. Skin is the largest organ in the body. It is made up of 70 percent water, and drinking plenty of fluids every day is one of the best ways to prevent the skin from drying out and wrinkling. I recommend that you don't drink water thirty minutes before or three hours after eating, however. Water can prevent the natural oils and minerals in food from getting into the lymphatic system,

which carries these nutrients to the joints, skin, and hair where they are needed.

3. Make sure your diet is rich in nucleic acids; chlorophyll; vitamins C, E, and niacin; and the minerals selenium and silicon. To promote circulation, exercise regularly. Nucleic acids help slow down the "aging" of cells, including skin cells. Chlorophyll and Vitamin C help flush wastes out of the surface capillaries. Niacin expands the capillaries and increases blood circulation to the skin, removing wastes and bringing nutrients. Similarly, exercise cleanses the skin pores and enhances circulation. I will explore the impact of nutrition and exercise on your total health later.

4. When you wash your face, use a mild soap and warm water. Follow with ten rinses of cold water to close the pores and hold the moisture in.

5. To cleanse the skin and exercise the muscle structure of the face, I recommend the "honey pat." Apply hot (not steaming) towels to the face, then cold towels (not ice cubes or crushed ice) to get the circulation going. Then pour a little raw honey into a saucer and apply it to your face (after drying the skin with a towel). Avoid the areas surrounding the eyes. Let the honey set for two to five minutes, then begin patting your face slowly with both hands, letting the sticky honey draw the skin out until it "snaps back" naturally. This tones the face muscles and cleans clogged pores. Pat the face for about five minutes, then remove the honey with a wash cloth and warm water.

A WORD FOR THE MEN

One of the most important things I've learned is that the "homeliest" man in the world can be popular and attractive to men and women alike, if he is outgoing, energetic, not self-conscious, friendly, and has a good sense of humor. Can you believe that how you look to others is strongly influenced by how they feel about you? Can you believe that how others feel about you is strongly influenced by how you feel about yourself?

What you are in your innermost self, you really are. Don't settle for less. If you are naturally attractive to women, your looks can be a blessing or a curse, depending on the kind of person you are underneath the attractive exterior. If you aren't much on looks, you'll benefit from your efforts to try harder, to make the best of what you have.

Most men want to look good to other men as well as women, so they can feel accepted and approved by their peers as well as appearing attractive to the opposite sex. I don't know of a single man who doesn't enjoy a compliment from other men, such as, "you really look sharp, George." Nor do I know of a single man who doesn't like being looked at or admired by women.

The heart of being attractive, for men, is liking yourself. When you can gratefully accept the gifts, talents, interests, abilities, physical characteristics, and looks nature has given you, and be satisfied with them, you're on your way to being accepted and attractive to others. This acceptance has much to do with self-confidence.

Why do I keep mentioning self-confidence? Think about it for a moment. If you don't appreciate and feel good about yourself, how can you expect women to feel good about you?

Women evaluate a man's looks, but they are really attracted most by a man's actions. How a man acts reveals his level of self-confidence. Call it "good vibrations," "chemistry," "dynamic magnetism," or whatever you want, the masculine personality is always one of the first things a woman becomes interested in—if you are her type. The masculine personality is something a woman senses quickly and intuitively.

Who you are is also expressed through your level of friendliness, the sparkle in your eyes, your hair, clothes, posture, tone of voice, your level of enthusiasm about life, the interest shown toward others, and what you talk about.

LOVE: THE BEST COSMETIC

At the beginning of this chapter, I indicated that beauty is more than skin deep because our bodies were made to serve as a means of expressing the soul-life given to each of us. The soul-life consists of thought, emotions, and will (or purpose), plus specific gifts, talents, and abilities. I believe that no person can be truly beautiful unless he or she is healthy and fulfilled through love, including sexuality. Love—really caring for someone outside yourself—is absolutely necessary to maintain a positive attitude, good health, and attractiveness. In this sense, love may be the most amazing "cosmetic" of all.

Part Two
SEX

Chapter Eight
Secrets of the Glands

You couldn't wink and really mean it without the help of your endocrine glands. I don't mean to take the fun out of flirtation by stating the importance of the glands that way. Neither do I intend to overemphasize the science behind love and sex. Nevertheless, you may want to know how the glands control sex. I believe that you can still have fun with this knowledge.

While the brain initiates sexual feelings, any follow-up sexual activity would be impossible without the aid of the endocrine glands, which nourish, sustain, and activate the human reproductive system. In a sense, these glands support our capacity and desire to love, as well as our capacity and desire to reproduce sexually. Love and sex would only be words without glands to give them life, energy, urgency, and feeling.

The brain controls or regulates the body by sending electrical messages through the nervous system, much the same as a telephone center sends out messages through its lines. A single message can be sent on "one line" to a single muscle or organ, or a general message can be sent to all body tissues. Some parts of the nervous system can stimulate or inhibit glandular functioning, and the brain exercises a great deal of control over the glands.

The endocrine system, in contrast to the brain and nervous system, operates by releasing chemical messengers from specific glands. These chemical messengers, called hormones, enter and circulate in the bloodstream. Although they are exposed to a great many kinds of tissues as they travel through the bloodstream, each hormone is designed to stimulate only certain types of activity with a certain type (or types) of tissue. Glands can trigger or inhibit nerve impulses, just as nerves can trigger or inhibit hormone release.

Our glands are the treasure chest from which sexual delight and satisfaction are drawn. If the glands are inherently weak, we must take better care of them to have a good life. Inherently weak glands are like a treasure chest in which very little reserve is kept, and we have to keep replenishing it. We have to feed the glands well all the time, using a proper diet. We have to have enough exercise and rest. We have to have the right attitude and avoid excess stress, since the thyroid, for example, is very sensitive to emotional shock and can easily become underactive.

Perhaps the best example of the interrelationship between nutrition, health, and glands is the hypothalamus. Linked by nerves to the nervous system and endocrine system, the hypothalamus permits both direct and indirect exchanges between glands and brain.

Because of the close relationship between brain function and glandular function, anything that disrupts normal brain activity (such as chronic job stress) will affect the glands, starting with the most inherently weak glands. Therefore, we have to learn to handle or eliminate our problems without breaking down the glands.

Not all endocrine glands are directly related to sexual functioning. But all are indirectly related to the sex life, as much as they are to a person's overall health. While hormones are released in minute amounts, they are extremely powerful in their action. Let's take a look at the names of our endocrine glands, their locations, the hormones they produce, and their functions in the body.

TYPES OF HORMONES

Endocrine system hormones affect—among other things—our moods, behavior, immunity, metabolism, blood sugar, rate of healing, and sexual and reproductive performance. There are three categories of hormones produced by the endocrine glands: *polypeptide hormones, steroid hormones,* and *prostaglandins.*

Polypeptide Hormones

Many polypeptide hormones act as "messenger" hormones to trigger the release of other hormones such as the sexual hormones *estrogen, testosterone* in males, and *progesterone* in females; or act directly in the brain as neurotransmitters (nerve transmitters).

Major Endocrine Glands and Their Functions

Pituitary Gland (Master Gland of Endocrine System). Located in base of brain. Regulates pre-adult growth, sexual development, fertility, and other glands in endocrine system.

Thyroid Gland. Located in throat. Controls metabolism of entire body by regulating energy production and oxygen. Also regulates blood calcium.

Pineal Gland. Located at base of brain. Mystery gland. May affect ovarian secretion, menstrual cycle, and stimulate adrenals to produce the sex hormone aldosterone.

Parathyroid Glands. Located in the thyroid. Regulate calcium and phosphate in the blood by dissolving these elements from bone when needed.

Adrenal Glands. Located above kidneys. Regulate carbohydrate metabolism, healing, heart rate, blood pressure, blood sugar, water, and electrolyte recovery; male and female sex hormones.

Prostate Gland. Located in men only, below urinary bladder. Produces fluid to protect sperm.

Islets Of Langerhans. Located in the pancreas. Regulate blood sugar level by storing excess and increasing cell sugar use.

Thymus Gland. Located behind breastbone, between lungs. Aids immune system function by producing special cells called T-cells.

Ovaries. Located in female pelvic area. Produce sex hormones, regulate menstrual cycle, maintain pregnancy, prepare for lactation, site of egg production.

Testes. Located in male pelvic area. Produce sex hormones. Site of sperm production.

The actions of these hormones are very powerful but only on specific tissues for which they are designed. They work by improving or changing the metabolism of these tissues. The actions are often interrelated, with one hormone triggering the release of another, this leading to another, and so on.

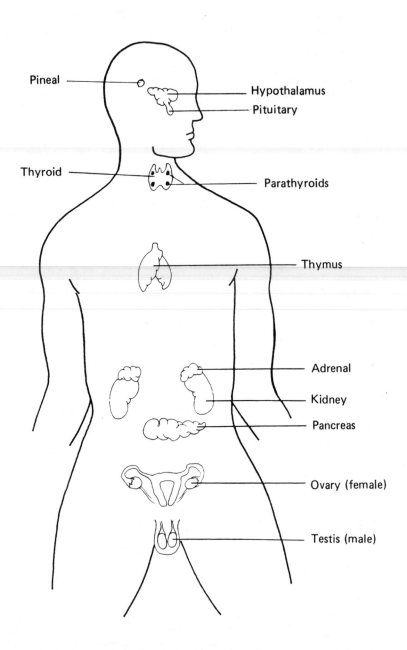

The Human Endocrine Glands

Common Hormones

Hormone	Gland	Function
HRF	Hypothalamus	Pituitary control
ACTH, Growth Hormone	Pituitary	Sexual development
TSH	Pituitary	Thyroid stimulation
Thyroxin	Thyroid	Metabolism regulation
Parathormone	Parathyroids	Blood calcium regulation
Thymosin	Thymus	Immune defense
Glucocorticoids	Adrenals	Stress resistance

For example, the hypothalamus of the brain, just above the pituitary, monitors activity levels of various tissues of the body. When the metabolism drops too low, the hypothalamus releases a polypeptide hormone called TRF that goes directly to the pituitary and triggers the release of a second hormone called TSF (thyroid stimulating factor). The TSF acts only on the thyroid gland, signaling it to release another chemical called thyroxine until the metabolic rate increases to normal.

Steroid Hormones

Steroid hormones are fatty-based substances with a cholesterol-type nucleus, such as the hormones made in and secreted from the adrenal cortex, ovaries, or testes. These include not only the sex hormones such as progesterone, estrogen, and testosterone but also steroids that influence carbohydrate-, fat-, and protein metabolism. These steroids help the body handle stress and assist in resisting infection. In recent years, steroids that assist in weight gain and muscle building have created controversy when it was discovered that athletes have used them illegally. Steroid additives to livestock feed have been outlawed in the United States because they increase the risk of cancer in those who eat the meat.

Prostaglandins

Prostaglandins are made from fatty acids. Unlike hormones they are not produced in the endocrine glands but in the specific areas of the body where they are used by local cells. Some research suggests that certain prostaglandins are activated by other hormones that enter the tissue area. The prostaglandins probably cause the actual tissue change. Many different kinds of prostaglandins have been discovered. Research on prostaglandins has shown that they affect the raising and lowering of blood pressure, bring relief from pain, and stimulate the production of steroids.

WHAT MAKES GLANDS SEXY?

Endocrine glands affect human sexuality not only in specific, sex-linked, ways but also by the creation of an active, healthy, energetic environment inside the human body. As I have often heard from my patients, sex is meaningless to someone with poor physical health or no energy. You have to have energy to jump for joy.

Enjoyable sex is impossible without enough energy to actively "play" with your partner, and available energy is often determined by glands not directly related to our sexual functions. Lack of energy may be the result of hypothyroidism (low thyroid function) or hypoglycemia (low blood sugar) because of problems with the Islets of Langerhans in the pancreas. Both are endocrine malfunctions.

Endocrine glands are interdependent. When one becomes underactive, the others are affected. Though the strong glands support the weak glands, the stronger all endocrine glands are, the better and more enjoyable sexual responsiveness will be. Here, once again, we encounter the principle that it is best to take care of the entire system—the endocrine system in this case—instead of treating an individual gland or glandular imbalance.

When the glandular system is out of balance, the brain and body are affected—and physical problems of one kind or another emerge as a result. Behavioral or mental problems, such as violence or depression, may also result. The list of endocrine gland-related diseases and problems is too long for this book. The point is that we need to take good care of our glands in order to have good sex lives.

Proper nutrition and positive attitude are critical to attaining a good love life and a good sex life. It is not difficult to throw the endocrine system out of balance. It can be done with fad reducing diets, junk-food, or unbalanced diets. It can be done with drugs or alcohol. It can be done through chronic emotional extremes such as constant bitterness, anger, resentment, jealousy, or hate. It can be done with stress.

MALE GLANDULAR FUNCTION

At puberty, the pituitary gland releases follicle stimulating hormone (FSH) and interstitial cell-stimulating hormone (ICSH) which set in motion the process of sexual maturation and preparation for reproduction. FHS stimulates the testes to begin to make sperm. ICSH triggers the production of testosterone. Soon after, the lowered voice and the narrow-hipped, broad-shouldered, male body begin to appear.

This change in hormonal activity is accompanied by dramatic and somewhat unsettling emotional changes. Alterations in blood chemistry influence the way a young man perceives himself, other men, and women. Generally a young male may take a couple of years to adjust to the internal and external changes through which he is going.

Both personality and physique are affected by the glandular changes that accompany puberty. As men grow older, the predominant presence of the male hormone, testosterone—and the relatively lower amounts of the female hormones, estrogen and progesterone—may lead to balding and increased risk of heart disease. The prostate and bulbourethral glands make chemical substances that keep sperm active and fertile. The testicles produce sperm and hormones, particularly testosterone, which determine secondary male characteristics (such as a muscular body, deep voice, and hairy chest). Testosterone stimulates an increase in protein production, strengthens bones, broadens shoulders, and raises the general metabolism level.

FEMALE GLANDULAR FUNCTION

The lovely curves that men find so attractive among women are a direct result of the female hormones developed and released at puberty. At a signal from the brain, these hormones are released from the pituitary gland. By stimulating production of estrogen and progesterone in the ovaries they prepare the female reproductive system to bear children. Estrogen signals developmental changes such as enlarging breasts, widening of the pelvis, the growth of pubic hair, and the beginning of the menstrual cycle. Progesterone works with estrogens to prepare the endometrium (the inner lining of the uterus) for the fertilized egg implantation and the breasts for milk secretion.

Female sex hormones promote the soft, clear skin and the layer of fat beneath the skin that produces the soft, feminine curves. They also protect women from cardiovascular disease until menopause, the time when fertility and menstruation end and hormone levels change dramatically.

It is also important to acknowledge that, because of monthly cyclic changes in a women's body, her mind and emotions respond differently than a man's. At times, a woman may seem to be extra-sensitive emotionally—quick to laugh; quick to cry. Pregnancy, menstruation, and menopause among women are all accompanied by significant hormonal shifts that affect the emotions and behavior. (Recent research has shown that men are affected by hormone release cycles as well as women.)

WE ARE AS YOUNG AND SEXY AS OUR GLANDS

"You're as young as your glands," goes the old saying. The glands have a natural cosmetic effect on our entire being. Only if our glands are healthy and functioning properly can we enjoy a fulfilling sex life. When our glands are working well and in balance, our skin, hair, and nails are more attractive. There's a spring in our step and a glow to our cheeks. We are more sensitive, bright, and happy.

Dr. Mark Gold of Friends Hospital in Philadelphia, Pennsylvania, has found that depression is often triggered by an underactive thyroid, which reduces the amount of the hormone *thyroxine* and produces changes in the brain. I feel the moping, depressed, downtrodden, behavior we see in many people—particularly the elderly—is due to glandular imbalance. We can't be well unless we are happy, and we can't be happy unless we keep all of our glands healthy by feeding and caring for them properly. Happiness has been linked to a more effective immune system function and to the brain's increased production of *endorphins,* morphine-like chemicals associated with well-being. Endorphins are the brain's natural way of making us feel better all over; thus healthy glands and a healthy attitude are directly related.

Another key to good health and a fulfilling sex life is controlling the adrenal glands. One function of the adrenal glands is to release a hormone in times of danger that helps us to respond immediately by "fight or flight." The hormone is *adrenaline* (also called epinephrine), and its effect is extremely powerful. It increases the heart rate, raises blood sugar, constricts blood vessels,

Common Sources of Stress

Divorce or separation	Job change
Pregnancy	Unhappiness with job
Abortion	Moving
Hospitalization	PMS (Premenstrual Syndrome)
Sexually transmitted disease	Job promotion
Broken love affair	Jet lag
Marriage	Risk of job loss
Reconciliation	Purchase of home
Serious health problem	Brush with the law
Loss of job	Jail or prison sentence
Loss of close friend	Alcoholic mate
Sex problems	Drug addicted mate
Financial problems	Abusive mate

increases respiration, and stimulates the metabolism—in other words, it prepares the body for emergency action. Adrenaline also plays an important role in sexual arousal and performance.

The problem is that many kinds of stress (following chart), frustration, fear, shock, surprise, and anger can trigger a surge of adrenaline, and, if it is not worked off by physical exercise, adrenaline can be damaging to the body. The body is designed to "burn off" adrenaline by running or fighting—not to neutralize it when no physical action is called for.

Though some people seem to thrive on thrills and the fast life, their adrenal glands can't continue to counteract these types of self-imposed stress indefinitely. Glandular depletion—deficiency in needed nutrients following overwork—strikes the inherently weak glands first and reduces their activity level. This interferes with the absorption of nutrients and the elimination of wastes and makes the glandular tissue vulnerable to toxic buildup. Toxins, such as those from food additives, settle in weak, deficient, overworked glands—and before we realize what is happening, our sex and overall health are threatened.

Stress is the invisible health threat of our time—the greatest danger to our nerves, glands, and mental and physical health. Normally, glands and organs are well-regulated by a "feedback" loop where the action initiated by the hormone can be slowed and stopped. These processes "cooperate" with thousands of other physiological and chemical activities in the body to generate what we experience as well-being or good health. When stress begins to take its toll, however, health can take a quick downhill turn. A poor diet combined with a lack of exercise can make the problem even worse. Inflammatory problems such as allergies and arthritis increase, the immune system falters leaving us susceptible to all kinds of invaders, cells die, and the aging process accelerates. The glands and their hormones regulate the efficiency of many of the body's systems, including our sexual development, arousal, and function. It would seem that our glands effect control far above proportion to their size, and this is true. It is also true, however, that the glands have their master, probably the most remarkable creation in all of life's miracles—the human brain.

Chapter Nine
Sex is a Brain Child

Though science has discovered much about the way the human brain works, much remains to be learned. The human brain is the most complex physiological/neurological/electrochemical structure found among the animals. Because much is yet to be learned about the brain, it is important to view the existing body of knowledge on it as incomplete. This attitude aids us in being open to new theories about how the brain works. Many current theories about the brain may be proven in time. Still others are bound to be forthcoming.

Usually, the last thing we would think of in considering our love lives and sexual happiness is the brain. Yet I would not be exaggerating if I were to say that the brain is the most important organ in the sexual system. Why is this?

We know that the brain literally rules each muscle, gland, and organ in the body. If the brain does not first move, the body does not follow. If part of the body is not functioning correctly, the brain is always involved. Every part of the brain influences every other part of the body, just as each part of the body influences every other part of the body.

For example, if the sex center, located in the brain's hypothalamus, is underactive, so are the other brain centers. The emotions may be depressed. The appetite center may be less active. Our sexual center in the brain, and the sexual system (including the sex glands and hormones) affect the activity and health level of every other cell and tissue in the body.

The opposite is also true. When the activity level of any other part of the brain is affected, the sex center will also be affected. A poorly-functioning liver, pancreas, kidney, or bowel will affect the sexual system. It is therefore possible that a person could have a strong and vital sexuality which, if there were serious health problems elsewhere in the body, could be reduced to complete disinterest. The conclusion should be obvious: We can't just look to the health of the sex center in the brain and the sex system in the body. We must care for the whole person.

THE HUMAN BRAIN AND HOW IT CONTROLS SEX

The average person's brain is about the size of a softball; weighs 2 and three-quarter pounds; and consumes up to 25 percent of the blood's oxygen to perform its tasks. At any one time, 20 percent of the body's total blood supply is in the brain, an organ that represents only about two percent of the total body weight. The brain uses enormous amounts of blood sugar (glucose) to do its work. And, if either oxygen or glucose is cut off, brain cells begin to die within minutes.

The average brain contains 16 billion cells whose nerve signals crackle with electromagnetic energy, thousands of them speeding through the brain at once. Some of this electromagnetic energy creates what we call consciousness, while the rest directs thousands of involuntary body functions. Some of this energy appears to organize and sustain our memories; and much of it is devoted to learning and to organizing our sensory experience.

It is easy to see therefore, that if our brains are not working correctly, neither will much else in our bodies—or our lives, for that matter. Therefore, the first thing we have to take care of is the brain. Because if our brains are not in the mood for love or sex, the rest of us won't be either.

We find that the sex lives of humans differ from those of other animals. Animals have a cyclic pattern of mating, and they remain uninterested in sex outside those cyclic periods. But men and women can become passionately aroused almost any time, either by external or internal stimulation. Unlike animals, humans can choose when we want to express ourselves sexually.

In humans, sexual arousal is both neural and glandular, and the process of arousal always begins in the brain. The sex center in man is located in the hypothalamus, a small, twin-lobed part of the brain lying just above the midbrain structure. The interesting thing about the hypothalamus is that it is a major nerve "switchboard center," and as we have mentioned, it exerts a controlling influence on the pituitary gland, the master gland of the endocrine system.

All five senses may take part in human sexual arousal. The visual sense appears to be the strongest initial agent of excitement, and I want you to notice the word "excitement." If there is no emotional response to seeing a member of the opposite sex, there will be no arousal. Granted, not everyone "turns us on." But the person who does will be found first by sight. After visual contact, either *hearing* or scent comes next in line. A person's voice can be an attractive force. So can the *smell* of a nice perfume or aftershave lotion. Scientists say that smell is one of the primordial attractive factors in the sex life of man. The sense of *touch*, seldom involved in the initial focus of attention, is the most intimate of the senses and the most arousing. Perhaps this is why during the early stages of a relationship even a touch of the hands can bring tingles or goosebumps to the person being touched. The sense of *taste* is involved through kissing, and this can be a wonderful sensory experience. Of course, the sense of touch is also involved in kissing. (For a detailed look at how the five senses influence the brain and sex, see the next chapter.)

As the five senses are involved, the emotions are aroused, the glands are stimulated, and the nervous system is engaged. The nerves send messages to the nerve plexus at the base of the spine, which relays these messages to the pelvic nerves. Tissues begin to swell with blood, the adrenal glands release adrenalin, the heart beats faster, the breathing rate increases, and the sex glands secrete fluids.

In this way, we come to view sex as a "conversation" between the body and mind. Instead of words, the communication is conducted with chemicals and nerve impulses.

Initially, as sex interest turns to arousal, sensory nerve impulses (sight, sound, smell, taste, touch) travel to the hypothalamus which signals the medulla, the *limbic system*, and the pituitary gland to get to work.

The medulla signals the lungs to take in more oxygen and the heart to beat more rapidly. The limbic system, centered in the midbrain, becomes "electrified" as the level of pleasure rises; and its vibratory intensity at the time of orgasm is quite powerful. From the limbic system, a brain chemical called phenylethylamine is released, a pleasure-producing chemical which, in lower levels, is responsible for feelings of "falling in love." Another chemical, called LHRH (luteinizing hormone releasing hormone), released by the hypothalamus, triggers the pituitary release of the sex-gland stimulating hormones but also stimulates the brain directly to produce sexual arousal and excitement.

In men, the pituitary-stimulated release of adrenalin, and a neurotransmitter called acetylcholine, are necessary for erection and orgasm. In both men and women, the pituitary's release of the hormone oxytocin (a polypeptide hormone) apparently initiates the involuntary vibrations of the pelvis that accompany orgasm.

Prior to orgasm, as sexual excitement mounts, people become more or less oblivious to pain and discomfort and their sense of time is distorted. As the body's messages to the mind become more frequent and more intense, the pleasure center of the brain begins to take over, and intense awareness of pleasure seems to blot out awareness of oneself and the other person. At the point of orgasm, up to 25 percent of the body's oxygen may be expended.

While powerful, short-lived chemicals and nerve-stimulated events take part in sexual arousal, orgasm, and pleasure, a longer-term brain chemical is probably involved in more stable relationships. As I have mentioned, morphine-like brain chemicals called endorphins act to develop long-term pleasure in the relationship between two people.

All of this begins from a little "tickle" in the healthy brain. When the brain is fatigued, emotionally overwrought, or depleted of key nutrients, these events may not occur. Impotence or frigidity are signs that something needs to be taken care of in the brain, body, or mind. Such symptoms are basically protective mechanisms to warn us against further chemical depletion or further mental and emotional exhaustion.

BRAIN "SEX-BLOCKERS"

There are several ways we can interfere with good brain function and diminish our sexuality. If you don't eat the right foods, the brain will not be nourished well enough to keep you full of vitality. If you don't have enough iron in the blood to foster the growth of red blood cells that carry the necessary oxygen, the brain is forced to slow down. If you get plenty of good food and are taking in plenty of oxygen, it won't do you much good if your circulation is so poor that not enough blood gets to the brain. Usually poor circulation comes from lack of exercise. Since the blood must be pumped "uphill" against gravity to get to the brain, exercise is necessary at any age to prevent what we call brain anemia.

There are other common ways we abuse and mistreat our brains. We overwork it in high-stress jobs. We wear it down with a turbulent emotional life. We drain it with negative thoughts and attitudes. These conditions wear out the brain just as much as lack of oxygen or nutrients do. In fact, overworking or abusing the brain depletes it of needed nutrients, reducing its capacity to respond to the body's needs. An overworked, depleted brain cannot love, and the sexual appetite is diminished.

Indeed, we find that stress is the most insidious enemy of the brain. It creeps in as stealthily as a cat in tennis shoes, robs us of vitality, and leaves the nervous system and brain depleted. Stress is one of the main contributors to fatigue and toxemia, as well. These are also enemies of the brain.

Stress works on the hypothalamus; creates nerve acids, interferes with digestion, assimilation and elimination; and tends to break down inherently weak organs and systems in the body. Stress distorts emotional response, downgrades motivation levels, and destroys the sex life. I believe the latter is caused by the multiple environmental effects of stress, but pituitary imbalance and hormonal insufficiency, both controlled by the brain, are certainly among the most important physiological causes of loss of sex interest.

Fatigue is similar to stress in that it reduces the efficiency of digestion, assimilation, and elimination; increases the level of nerve acids and metabolic wastes in the body; and reduces the level of neural and glandular function. Tired people don't want romance, love, and sex—they want rest. And, they need rest.

Toxemia, an excess of toxic materials in the blood and lymphatic system, is often a consequence of chronic stress or chronic fatigue, but it may also be caused by a poor diet, overuse of drugs, pollution in the environment, exposure to chemicals in the workplace, or even chronic constipation. The thyroid gland responds to toxemia by lowering the available body energy, and the brain responds by a kind of nervous fearfulness, insecurity, loss of will, and confusion.

Toxemia of a different kind can be produced by food addictions—not only to substances like alcohol and caffeine but also eggs, wheat, milk, and chemical components like gluten from a number of grains. Chronic food allergies are linked to food addiction when people begin to crave the "body feeling" they get from eating certain foods. Food allergies often have a "target organ" that they affect the most, as wheat allergy affects the intestine.

The brain can become the organ most seriously affected by some foods. The result can be "recognizable mental or behavior changes," says Dr. Richard Mackarness, author of *Eating Dangerously*. Temper problems, irritability, depression, unhappiness, fear, nervousness, nightmares, and loss of interest in sex can occur.

Brain Sex Blockers

Problem	Cause	Solution
Brain fatigue.	Stress, overwork leads to depletion of brain nutrients faster than they can be replaced.	Rest, recreation, nature walks, exercise.
Anemia.	Not enough iron-rich blood reaching the brain.	Eat foods high in iron and B vitamins, liver, green leafy vegetables, eggs, Brewer's yeast.
Toxins in blood.	Body wastes, drugs, food additives, and environmental pollutants.	Short-term fasting, eat only pure, natural foods.
Organic disease.	Hypothyroidism and glandular diseases.	See your physician.
Sexual excess.	Body is robbed of lecithin and creative discipline.	Learn to channel your sexual energy.

HOW CAN WE KEEP OUR BRAINS HEALTHY?

The brain, like the rest of the body, is made up of chemical elements. But what we call the "mind" or "soul" is not material, not substance. We do not feed our souls with protein, fats, and carbohydrates—but with love, beauty, color, music, nature, light, and the proper expression of our unique purpose in life.

When we stop and think about it, all thoughts, feelings, and perceptions are expressed through the physical vehicle of the brain as vibrations, as electromagnetic impulses that generate an electromagnetic field of ultra-high frequency. I'm talking about the total effect of nerve impulses in the average brain. When these vibrations are in harmony, life and health are wonderful. When they are in conflict, the integrity of life and health is compromised.

The light that reaches the visual cortex is made of electromagnetic vibrations. The sounds that travel over the 27,000 auditory nerves to the brain are electromagnetic vibrations. Our thoughts and emotions generate electromagnetic vibrations. How these vibrations harmonize or conflict with one another determines the quality of our lives, and it is through the quality of our lives that our relationships with others are determined.

One of the greatest differences between humans and animals is that humans can choose to change when their lives need improving. Animals need trainers to help change them. Of course, we have behavior modification techniques for people, too, but many people have managed to make great changes in their lives without paying psychologists to help them.

Many of my patients who considered sex as a mere performance were looking for some method of stimulating themselves physically, some kind of pill. I had to tell them sex starts in the mind, in the brain. That's where we have to start.

Keep in mind that the hypothalamus, where the sex center is located, receives messages from the sensory nerves, the glands, and organs. There are many "wires" that plug into our sex switchboard to influence our sexual behavior, and at the present time we know very little about the relative importance of each wire and its relationship to others. What we do know is sufficient to indicate that healthy brain function is crucial to the love and sex life of humans.

We all seek vitality. We all want to feel wonderful as much as we can; and our love lives, our sex lives, seem to be essential to this vitality, the feeling we have when life feels wonderful. Love and sex seems to provide one means of releasing the life force involved in all creative enterprises—from thoughts to business.

This life force flows through the universe. It's in the sunshine, it's in the growth of plants and flowers, it's in the laughter of babies, and it's in the food we eat. If we choose the right foods,

Exercises for Mind/Brain Health

Here are some mind exercises designed to improve minds and lives at the same time. Concentrate your attention on each phrase as you repeat it, believing that it is true.

- Every time I think, I open a channel for the higher expression of my life and my love.

- I know that loving thoughts are healing thoughts, and every day my body grows healthier and stronger.

- Love is the strongest force for good in the universe, and I am filled with love.

- I believe I will achieve a whole, pure, and natural lifestyle and a stronger, healthier more responsive body.

- My sex life is as beautiful as the path I have selected in life, and every day in every way, my path is getting better and better.

- I will think only those things which I desire to manifest in my life, whatever is clean, whatever is pure, whatever is good, whatever is beautiful.

- I know my body will express what my mind decides, and my resolve is to love more, to raise the level of my sex life, and to be a stronger, more energetic, more helpful person.

- This very day I affirm I will be:
  —calm and happy,
  —full of peace and joy,
  —patient and kind,
  —forgiving and full of good will,
  —confident and trusting,
  —full of faith and faithful,
  —wise and considerate,
  —able to handle any situation,
  —free to love and be loved.

we release the maximum life force. If we choose the wrong foods, we can develop sickness or disease instead of health.

Sickness and disease are always accompanied by a lowering of the life force, a lowering of available energy. When this happens, the sex life is one of the first casualties because the brain switches all circuits to conserve energy in the body so that available energy can be used to restore the body to health. When the sex life is shut down, the life force and energy level drop another notch.

Consequently, we find that every health problem affects the sex life and every sex problem affects health. The two are interrelated, and the brain determines the relationship. Because the human brain is so crucial to sex, and health in general, we need to make deliberate and concentrated efforts to keep the brain sound. Fortunately, human beings can adapt, change their bad habits for good, and exercise the brain.

Chapter Ten
Sex and the Five Senses

While the brain and endocrine glands must be "turned on" for anyone to fall in love or be sexually aroused, we have to be aware of what turns on the brain and glands. This is why we need to look into the senses and the roles they play in love and sex. As defined briefly in Chapter Nine, the basic five senses are sight, hearing, touch, taste, and smell. All are important in human sexuality.

Sense organs allow us to respond to our environment which includes other people. When specialized cells associated with sense organs are stimulated, they send nerve impulses to the brain. Response to this stimulation comes from the brain and endocrine system. Our eyes respond to light waves, our hearing responds to sound waves, our taste buds respond to dissolved chemicals. Basically, all our senses are triggered by vibratory waves that are transformed and organized by the brain into sense experience. Each sense can work independently of the others or, more often, all the sensory apparatus can cooperate to send a complex sexual message to the brain.

It is interesting to note that each sense has its own nuances. The sense of touch, for example, is not a single sensation. We feel the difference between touch, pressure, pain, heat, and cold. We feel sensations of movement, including falling, whirling, and speed. We feel such common sensations as hunger, thirst, nausea, and sexual desire, which are generated in the brain.

In addition to the sense of touch, smell plays an important role in the reproduction of many species of animals. The sounds of birds and cries of animals in their natural habitats are often associated with mating. Vision is probably the primary sense affecting at least the initial stage of sexual awareness among men and women.

To understand the sensory experience of the average human being, we need to understand that our brains influence how we interpret our experience. We don't all regard the same works of art as beautiful, do we? We don't all like the same music, do we? This is because our individual "tastes" or priorities in sensory experience are "screened" or sorted out in advance in the brain on a scale that ranges from "most desirable" to "least desirable."

DO WE SEE WHAT WE WANT TO SEE?

Some people are blind, others see only shades of gray (and are color-blind), and still others see most but not all colors. Still others' vision is disturbed to the point where they see patches or blurs of color or light, but not the clear, well-defined, colorful world that most of us see.

We hear people saying, "They don't see eye-to-eye." That goes for lovers as well as others who may disagree, but it is more important for lovers and marriage partners to agree than others. Harmony in relationships depends on healthy, accurate, perceptions—as well as good sense and wisdom in the interpretation of those perceptions.

I believe that color and beauty play an important role in the lives of normally-sighted people. Vision is important. (I do believe visually-handicapped people have compensating sensitivities.)

Nearly everyone has colors they regard as favorites and other colors they simply don't care for. When a man or woman sees the colors he or she loves worn by a member of the opposite sex, the colors attract attention and create a favorable response. It may also be the combination of colors that makes the impression.

When a person is wearing his favorite colors, he tends to be more alive and expressive, more confident and outgoing. Some women feel more feminine wearing certain colors, and also more attractive. Women have their favorite shades of eye shadow and makeup that help them to enhance their natural skin, hair, and eye color.

Now I can't with fairness say that all men and women dress to impress members of the opposite sex, but I believe many do. And when we stop and think about it, we find that people of certain personality types tend to be more attracted to some colors than others. This means that the color of the clothes we wear draws the attention and favor of certain personality types to us, while possibly repelling others.

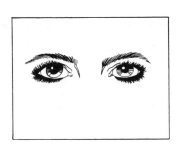

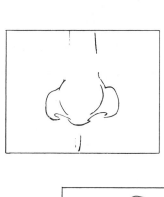

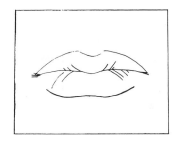

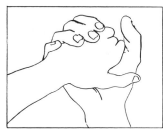

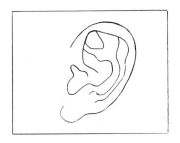

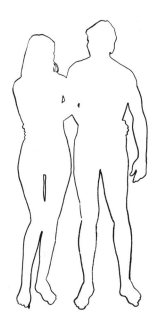

Sex and the Five Senses.
The five senses play an
important role, both
individually and collectively,
in love and sexual relationships.

We need to realize that certain colors have specific effects on people, as found in color research. Comments such as, "He painted the town red," or "I've got the blues," or "You're looking in the pink today," have a basis in fact. Red is a sexually provocative color and has been shown to be an arterial stimulant. Light blue has a calming effect on most people but can become depressing if a person stays around it too long. Royal blue brings out the noble qualities in people, as does purple of a rich hue. Yellow is said to act on the nerves, uplifting all systems and raising the mood level. Orange, a combination of red and yellow, stimulates the blood, brain and nerves, elevates moods, and, in some hues, stimulates humor and laughter. Green is a tranquilizing, healing color. Grass and trees are nature's color therapy to man. Pink has been used in prisons and mental institutions to calm violent tendencies. Violet is a healing color, one that uplifts the soul and encourages spiritual tendencies. White light contains all the colors of the rainbow and is traditionally a symbol of mourning, of death. Brown represents decay, and the color gray conveys the sense of white's intensity subdued with the addition of a measure of black.

When we select clothing, our best colors are those that complement the hair, skin, and eyes. The effects of colors and color combinations on us differ depending on the size and shape of the person wearing them—whether he or she is tall or short, of ample proportions, average or slender.

We need to be conscious of how the colors of clothes and makeup affect those around us. Men are generally aroused more when women wear reds, oranges, and shades of purple. Men take a lower key, friendlier stance (with fewer sexual overtones) when women wear blues, yellows, and whites. Of course, there are some women who appear sexy in virtually anything they wear, while others can carry that sweet, innocent look even in a scarlet dress. These examples are of a person's manner and style overpowering the effects of the clothing color.

Women, while more color-conscious than men, may not respond sexually to the colors of men's clothing in the same ways as men do to the colors of women's clothing. This is because men's suits are manufactured in a relatively narrow color range—generally black, gray, brown, and blue. That's why it is difficult to tell how women respond to men wearing suits. It is likely that women respond more to the facial features, physical build, manners, and personality than to the suit color.

Like color, light has been shown to affect our moods. In fact, researchers have found what may be a link between light and sexuality in humans. They have established that neurochemical channels connect light receptors in the retina of the eye with parts of the brain that regulate human sexuality, particularly the pineal gland. This research, however, is only in the beginning stages.

Based partly on this data, I believe adequate sunlight is necessary for an active, healthy sex life. It is also evident to me that particular colors, and probably particular frequencies of light, stimulate sexual feelings while others tend to depress sexual feelings. Dark colors make a person appear more dominant while light colors and pastels are more associated with mild, more submissive personalities. Highly-stimulating colors raise the energy level and mental alertness, while a combination like brown and blue creates a more relaxed, low-energy mood.

Be wise in what you wear—and tasteful. Consider what effect you want to produce on people, and why. If you want to raise the excitement level of a person who is special in your life, that's one thing, but if you are going somewhere where you want to communicate clearly with people, avoid "arousal colors." For instance, women executives should probably avoid wearing sexually-provocative colors to business functions because they might spend too much time warding off unwanted approaches by men!

In conclusion, light, color, and beauty, in general, are soul foods, nutrients for the mind. We need the vibrations they generate to keep certain brain and nerve centers activated, so that the soul qualities we have been given can be properly expressed in our path of life.

FLIRTATION

Unlike clothing colors, which "broadcast" their effects to all who see them, the use of flirtation is an art which can be controlled and directed for the visual benefits of specific people. Though the essence of successful flirtation is visibility, its nature should be low-key and unobtrusive, because its purpose is to secure the attention of just one person whom you want to know better. Women are generally better at flirting than men. One of the oldest acts of flirtation is when a woman crosses her legs as a man she likes is approaching.

Either sex can flirt with the eyes, but the method is different for the two sexes. A woman should glance at a man whose attention she wants to attract, then drop the glance right away when the man sees it. A man should hold his gaze in eye contact with the woman he is interested in, then smile. Don't break eye contact; and if the woman smiles back, go talk with her.

Men tend to be attracted by womens' arm and hand gestures as long as they aren't too nervous or wild. Women should use hand- and arm gestures that show the palms up, wrists exposed.

Granted, a healthy person who wears simple, attractive cloth- ing and acts himself or herself will seldom have to use artificial means of appearing attractive. But it's often fun to highlight and enhance our favorable qualities.

THE SEXIEST SOUNDS

Sex and sound have been linked as long as birds have sung to attract mates. But among humans, music and conversation seem to be among the most preferred ways that two persons can ap- proach intimacy once interest has been established by an initial visual check.

Since the era of the medieval troubadours, music has been associated with romance. Today, concerts are popular with lovers of all ages, since music has a way of enhancing and sweetening the savor of love. But the types of music to which we listen can affect our moods and behavior. I feel it is important to recognize that the wilder, more frenzied types of music tend to appeal to the baser instincts and emotions, and may create disharmony in the electro- magnetic fields of the brain. "Music soothes the savage beast," goes the old saying. In our time, there is also music that seems to generate savagery in ordinary people—whether sexual savagery or the tendency toward violent, bizarre behavior.

On the other hand, there are musical compositions that lift the soul to heights of love, that stir the higher emotions, that bring out the best in a person. There is romantic music, instrumental or vocal, that can turn an ordinary evening into heaven—with the right person's company.

Like so many things in life, we can choose what music we want to allow our ears to transmit to the brain, and we should choose the kind of music that stimulates or enhances peace, love, and harmony.

SMELL AND TASTE

The olfactory (smell) center of the brain is connected to the hypo-thalamus, and research has shown that it plays a part in human sexuality. Over 25 percent of those with olfactory problems lose interest in sex as a result. Not long ago, scientists discovered the apocrine glands at the roots of hair follicles. Underarm- and geni-tal hair picks up and holds the scent of the apocrine glands, which is believed to influence the choice of mate or lover. An experi-ment at the University of North Carolina showed that when syn-thetic vaginal scent was applied to the skin of young couples, they made love more often than before.

As we have mentioned, pheromones, once thought to affect insects only, are now known to affect human beings. Pheromones from men's bodies can stimulate their female sex partners to be more fertile, more regular in their menstrual cycles, and to have a milder experience with menopause. Women with long or short menstrual cycles tend to regularize after regularly inhaling men's pheromones, particularly if they have intercourse once a week. Women are also influenced by one another's pheromones, in the sense that women who share the same apartment often begin to menstruate at the same time after a few months. From perfumes to pheromones, odors are undeniably important in the process of human sexual attraction.

Taste, on the other hand, would seem to have a less direct relationship to sexual attraction—perhaps chiefly through kissing. Certainly taste can heighten the pleasures of sexual intimacy.

TOUCH

As we pointed out earlier, touching, caressing, cuddling, and holding are among the most important "bonding agents" in any relationship, whether of parent-child, husband-wife, or boy-friend-girlfriend. Touching sensations provide the "glue" that helps create a deeper sense of security and satisfaction in the relationship.

Most adults, according to the experts, still don't hold one an-other enough. A survey sent out by Ann Landers to thousands of women all over the United States showed that most of them, at any given time, would rather be cuddled than made love to. Men often misunderstand the need for touching, not only in their wives but themselves. Men need to be touched and held, too.

Caressing is particularly important in leading up to love making, and it is often neglected by men who are in a hurry to satisfy an urgent sexual drive. The problem is they are depriving their wives—and themselves, too—of a great deal of pleasure. Women take longer to warm up and become sufficiently aroused for joyful lovemaking, and they are often unable to respond with enthusiasm and excitement until reaching that stage. It takes a good deal of touching and caressing to get there.

In countries such as Italy, Spain, and France, people ordinarily touch more than they do in countries such as the United States and in Scandinavia. These European men hug and stand talking with an arm over another man's shoulders. Heterosexual men may greet one another with a kiss on the mouth or cheek. In these countries, no one considers this unusual behavior. This type of behavior is not generally socially-acceptable in the United States. As a result, I believe it is entirely possible that this type of "touch starvation" among United States men has contributed to the increase in homosexuality in this country in the last twenty years.

THE SENSES IN HARMONY

Consider the act of dancing for a moment, one of the most arousing public activities in our culture. When we dance, not only are bodies in contact (touch), they are in contact while swaying to a rhythm. The couple feels one another's body heat, skin, and perhaps even heartbeat. Each hears the other's breathing, whispered words of love, and the music in the background. They see each other and make frequent eye contact. Smell and taste can play their roles in this intimate—but public—exhibition of the power of the senses.

Similarly, though much more intimate, is human sexual expression itself. In the act of making love all the senses, the brain, and the spirit come together for timeless moments of ecstasy. But because the moments are so intense, so acute, the union of body, mind, and spirit depends on a healthy and absolute harmony.

Chapter Eleven
A Healthy, Natural Sexuality

Possibly the greatest problem we face today is that of coping with the staggering rate of change in our world. Traditional moral values cannot keep up with this rate of change. As a result, there exists much confusion around us in the areas of love, sex, and marriage. To many modern people, the question is, "How can a person have a healthy love life in an increasingly unhealthy world?"

WHAT IS A HEALTHY, NATURAL PHILOSOPHY TOWARD SEX?

I believe that Nature has been given to us as a model of life from which to learn. There is more wisdom in Nature than one person can discover in a thousand lifetimes. What can we learn about sex by observing Nature?

Nature is primarily interested in sex as a means to propagate future generations. For this reason, Nature has created a powerful urge to reproduce in all animals, including humans. Taking our cue from Nature, then, we conclude that the sex drive is not a built-in call to indulge in as much pleasure-oriented sex as possible with as many partners as possible. It is not our "animal nature" crying out to be released from all sexual restraint into a freedom of indulgence. It is, rather, Nature's tool to motivate us to reproduce for the survival of our species.

Among higher primates such as monkeys and humans, Nature has added another element to sex—intimacy. Nature has engineered the two to coexist in order to maintain the parental bond to nurture offspring who are relatively helpless for a relatively long period compared with other animals. With this example,

Nature teaches us that, between higher primates, sex has its place in the context of an intimate, ongoing relationship.

NATURE IS SURVIVAL-ORIENTED

By and large, Nature does not appear to endorse pleasure or oppose pain. Rather, Nature uses these sensations as means to an end. Nature tends to use pleasure to motivate animals to do things with a practical, life-oriented result. Likewise, Nature employs pain to motivate living things to avoid behavior that endangers life.

Nature's economy is based on survival-oriented traits, not on the luxury of self-indulgence and pleasure. Yet, unlike the other animals, man is capable of altering his own "nature" by creating an environment in which luxury and self-indulgence are the focus, not basic survival skills such as searching for food and water, avoiding death and injury, and mating to reproduce.

But though humans differ from the other animals in that they can alter their natural environments, Nature continues to react to our choices to protect life on our planet, regardless of whether we choose to ignore her life-protecting messages. Therefore, if we eat unwisely, we may attract disease and die before our natural time. If we use sex unwisely, we may develop emotional and psychological problems, disease, or, what can be worse, we can become "addicted" to it in such a way that all other aspects of our lives—work, exercise, rest, recreation, creativity, relationships, family life—become distorted and out of balance. These distortions lead to problems on a much larger scale. These are discussed in Chapter Thirteen: Our Modern "Disease."

WE EACH HAVE A DIFFERENT SEXUAL NATURE

If we consider what Nature has given to individuals, we find that some of us are highly sexual, some are moderately sexual, and some have little or no interest in sex. For some persons, having sex once a week can be too much. For others, ten times a week may not be too much. It depends on the person. Therefore, we need to respect our own natural limits and not try to keep up with some perceived "norm" in matters of sexuality. This "norm" does not exist.

To conclude, in nature, sex and sexuality play a small but essential role. Most animals mate solely for reproduction of their species. Nature is interested in its own self-perpetuation, not the pleasure of its creatures. Nature is not opposed to pleasure any more than it is opposed to pain. Its priorities are rather to use the life-patterns of all living organisms to create a rich and diverse tapestry of interrelated life on our planet.

FREEDOM AND RESPONSIBILITY

In some areas of the world, jackrabbits go through an eight-year population cycle. They reproduce so rapidly that, by about the seventh year, there is not enough food for all the jackrabbits. Because of this, they die by the millions, often from diseases that take over when their bodies are weakened by starvation. As a result, in the eighth year of this cycle, few jackrabbits are seen where thousands roamed the year before. These findings lead us to conclude that food supply and jackrabbit population are mutually limited by nature.

Similarly, humans in many parts of the world experience starvation or severe food shortage because of overpopulation. However, people in more prosperous and more technologically-advanced nations have been able to "trick" nature's process of mutual limitation. By using safe, effective forms of birth control, people in these countries have been able to achieve virtually unlimited sexual pleasure without unduly increasing population or depleting food supplies. So far, this "experiment" has succeeded in isolating sexual pleasure from its natural context of responsibility, thereby bestowing on it a relatively high social priority.

However, by harnessing sex to human convenience, the sex drive has created all sorts of complications on both large- and small scales.

Unwanted pregnancies result in thousands of abortions each year. Thousands more young people get married because they "have to"—and have unwanted children. Marriages end so often due to sexual infidelity that divorce has become commonplace.

It's bad enough that misuse of the sex drive has caused these changes that, in turn, have altered society by disrupting family life and confusing the nature of marriage. What's worse, misuse of the sex drive has, ultimately, generated a threat to life on earth by generating epidemics of sexually-transmitted diseases, the most deadly of which is AIDS.

The lesson that Nature teaches about sex, therefore, is to econ-omize—to value sex but not overvalue it; to enjoy sex but not to overemphasize it to such an extent that sex becomes an end in itself and thereby risks becoming a form of degradation; a means to destruction.

Nature aligns with basic economic philosophy in teaching us a fundamental principle: What is easily available becomes less valu-able. The true standard of nature is not found in the answer to the question, "Can life survive?" Rather it is found in the answer to the question, "Can life thrive?" Can it live well, without destroy-ing other communities of life around it? Perhaps society's attempt at harnessing sexuality to its most natural, practical use has re-sulted in the development of what we call moral values.

NOW IS THE TIME FOR CHANGE

Sometimes I think the word "morality" has gotten a bad reputa-tion. Perhaps it sounds too "goody-goody" and people don't take the concept of morality seriously any more. "Ethics" has had a similar decline in popularity. We therefore need a new language, or at least a few new power-packed words, to get people to sit up and listen long enough to realize that "right" and "wrong" are not retired—just temporarily unemployed.

Throughout much of the United States, jails and prisons are crammed to capacity with inmates sleeping on the floors. The AIDS epidemic has been estimated by some experts to become the single greatest threat to human life by the year 2000. Millions of men, women, and children are starving in Africa.

Can we agree that something needs to be changed?

I believe that we are seeing a good many sick people these days because we have lost sight of the usefulness of social and moral values. People don't know how to live right unless they have guidelines. And if you're not living right, you're living wrong. There isn't any neutral ground. I believe the problems we see all around us in our time show that we live in a sick society. A sick society will continue to produce more sick people until someone comes up with a cure or a way to reverse the process.

However, a degenerating social system is not automatically self-correcting. People have to do something to turn it around. We have become a nation of pleasure consumers, looking to other people to run things for us. The government can't do very much about moral degeneration. That's the people's business. But where are the people who will make it their business?

I believe we need a new philosophy which clearly identifies the dangers to human life and well-being today, and emphasizes preventive action, preventive education, and positive morality.

We need to start educating children in preschool about drugs, sex, and violence. We need to present a positive philosophy of life, a philosophy of right living, that children learn from a very early age. Children especially, but also the rest of us, need a "yardstick" we can use—a set of positive values—so that any idea, act, plan, or event can be measured to see if it's right or wrong. If it doesn't measure up to the yardstick, we shouldn't do it.

Children today need to be learning more than the "three R's"— reading, writing and arithmetic. They need to learn some new "R's," for instance, responsibility, relationships, renewal, and revitalization. A society in which moral standards are lax, such as ours, tends to breed unhappy, unhealthy people. Too many people think this world would be a much nicer place to live in if we just got rid of the rules and laws that keep people from having fun and doing what they want to do. But I believe that this is exactly opposite from the truth.

We do need rules, laws, and guidelines to point the way to a happy, healthy, productive life and to help prevent people from ruining their lives and the lives of others. For example, as a nutritionist I have found there are food laws we must follow to be physically healthy. Of course, many people live without following these basic nutritional rules, and these are the people who are filling up doctors' waiting rooms and hospital beds.

More than fifty-five years ago, I began my work in the health arts by emphasizing disease prevention within a philosophical context of holistic health. Holistic health emphasizes taking care of the whole body—body, mind, and spirit—rather than trying to eliminate disease symptoms. The strategy of "prevention" in the health arts is to teach people what they need to know to avoid disease and achieve their highest potential of well-being.

Similarly, there are social and moral laws we need to follow in order to live more productive, satisfying lives. If our society is somewhat "sick," then we must learn to treat the whole system, not just the symptoms. The abuse of alcohol and other drugs, widespread sexual promiscuity with little concern for the other person, crime, and hostility towards authority—all these can be viewed as symptoms of a more pervasive ethical and moral disease in our society.

The sad truth is, a pleasure-oriented society loses its ability to love because love cannot survive without responsibility and discipline. One of the main themes of this book is the need to love and be loved. Healthy, natural human sexuality should be nothing more, and nothing less, than an extension of this love, the fitting climax of the union of the body, mind, and spirit of one individual with that of another. When love for one's physical, mental, and spiritual self is combined with love for our fellow human beings, the result is more enthusiastic, fulfilled lives for all.

Chapter Twelve
Tender Sex

Perhaps the first step in making your life an example for the rest of society is to establish a truly loving relationship with another person. Of course there are many different kinds of relationships, and I am not saying that any one method will work for everyone. You and your partner should try to find what works best for you, but remember that sexual expression, when it is healthy, comes out of the love feeling, not the war feeling. There are many men— and perhaps even some women—who need to try a little tenderness. We find that tenderness is the true expression of love and by far the most gratifying approach in making the sex life meaningful.

WHAT THE SEX BOOKS MAY NOT TELL YOU

There are literally hundreds of books about sex out today, and their authors seem to be trying to outdo each other in sensational descriptions of positions and sexual acts that it would take two professional acrobats to get into. Even then I wonder if they would not have to see a chiropractor afterwards. Twenty years ago, many of these books could not have been published. I do not say they are bad. But I do believe they are creating three incorrect impressions.

The major error of most sex manuals is the extreme importance they place on sex, the overemphasis on its role in relationships. The second error is the overemphasis on technique. The third error of most sex manuals is their preoccupation with climax. Many, for example, encourage multiple orgasms in women or "TSO"—The Simultaneous Orgasm.

In my experience, the sex life is only 10 percent of a relationship. Love, friendship, consideration, courtesy, thoughtfulness, and a host of other priorities must be in their proper places before sex can be meaningful.

What the sex books fail to communicate is that too much explicit instruction can rob a couple of the delight that can come from exploration and discovery in the privacy of their own bedroom. While no book can even steal the ultimate mystery of the sexual expression and its beauty, too much instruction can make it seem like there is no mystery in sex, and it can generate the impression that good sex is more a mechanical skill than an art in a relationship.

TOUCHING SEX

Unless lovemaking is preceded by enough touching, it is seldom, if ever, fully satisfying—even if the final scenario is like an earthquake on the Fourth of July with bands playing and Roman candles exploding across the sky.

Touching includes a broad range of possibilities. It is nice if a couple learns some form of massage, so they can use it with one another. The whole body needs to be touched. A foot massage can be wonderfully relaxing. The arms and legs need to be kneaded, stroked, caressed. The head, neck, and scalp are relatively rich with sensitive nerve endings, and spending fifteen minutes on this area can seem like heaven to the one receiving the massage. Tension in many women is stored in the lower back, just above the kidneys, in the neck and in the trapezius muscles from neck to shoulder. Consider massaging these areas. In men, the neck, the trapezius muscles, and the muscles along the spine are often the storage areas for tension. In both sexes, the buttocks and the area where the thigh bone fits into its socket often need to be worked on. The whole body needs to be massaged, touched, and caressed.

Besides the kneading, pressure movements of massage, light stroking, and caressing are wonderful. Try touching with the finger tips, feather-light stroking with the fingers, soft slapping on the skin of the back, legs, feet, shoulders, and arms. A woman's breasts must be treated very gently, and her own desires in being touched there should be followed. Always communicate during massage to avoid bringing pain and discomfort to your partner. Tell each other what you like most and what you like least. Learn from each other.

After a time of touching and caressing, lovemaking is much more intimate, enjoyable, and satisfying. We find that when a couple is completely relaxed, it is sometimes well to join together in the sexual expression without thought of coming to a climax, and this is something that sex manuals seldom mention. There are occasions so intimate and romantic, in which two souls meet to share communion, that plunging toward a climax would spoil the tenderness of such a moment.

When Ann Landers found in her survey that 72 percent of all women would rather cuddle than have sex, I feel that women were expressing a starvation for intimacy and physical closeness, not a rejection of sex. The urgency and activity of a passionate sex drive can war against intimacy, turning lovemaking into a wrestling match. The urgent drive is nearly always the fault of the man who is in a hurry for the sexual expression. Many men fail to realize they are frustrating their own need for intimacy by hurrying through the sex act without slowing down to develop its full loveliness and meanings.

THE KAREZZA WAY

In the 1930s, a manuscript was circulated which described "Karezza," the principles of lovemaking used in the famed Oneida Community, founded by John Humphrey Noyes. Members of this community reported taking great delight and satisfaction in their love lives; and because this method seems appropriate to meet today's needs, I feel it is worth sharing.

The word Karezza means *caress* in Italian. This way of lovemaking emphasizes the spiritual and romantic values above plain sexuality, placing emphasis on the *person* rather than the act. Karezza recognizes that sex loses its intimacy in exact proportion as the partners focus on the act rather than each other. As the name implies, Karezza calls for a great deal of caressing and touching, which is what makes it so deeply satisfying.

Ideally, the couple who wishes to try Karezza should pick a time when they are alone, free of distractions for at least two hours, well rested, relaxed, and not in a hurry to do something else. The object is to concentrate entirely on love, joy, and harmony by avoiding urgency and passion-driven movements.

Each partner should be sensitive to the attractions of the other—the form, voice, touch, and fragrance. The intention of each should be to bless the other, to put the happiness' of the other person before one's own happiness.

The verbal part of Karezza may be the most difficult. American men, especially after a very few statements such as "You are really beautiful" and "I love you" are ready for the nonverbal part of lovemaking. But is is not that way in Karezza. Certainly men and women can both benefit from better bedroom communication.

Some persons are more reluctant or inhibited in talking about sex than others, and a few are unable to talk about it at all. But no matter how shy or reserved you are, you are going to have to learn to talk about making love—in the bedroom and in conversation before and after love. Otherwise, the other person is not going to learn what you like and what you don't like.

Rule Number One is, never say anything uncomplimentary about the other person before or during lovemaking. Because women take longer to warm up to experience the fullest enjoyment of their physical sensations, it is often up to the woman to encourage the man to take his time with a loving, slow preparation of kissing and touching before the main event begins.

It will help you to remember that you are putting the other person's happiness before your own. How many ways can you think of to compliment the other person? How many different expressions can you find to say, "I love you?" How can you express how much your partner means to you? What is it about your partner that you like and enjoy so much?

In the Karezza way, the talking is all done by the man, but I believe it can go both ways. The love partners may want to take turns talking or may agree that one person will do all the talking and caressing this time, and the other will do the talking and caressing the next time. Always spend time complimenting your partner on his or her body. It is not amiss during lovemaking to say, "Please slow down, darling—I want this to last a while longer." Learn to tell the one you love where and how you want to be touched. Everyone is different. Some like to play with considerable roughness, and some prefer soft, delicate touching. The important point to remember is we much communicate our desires in the right ways.

Don't say, "I hate it when you do that," say, "I want you to do it this way" or "I love it when you do this." If you are really bothered about something your lover is doing, you may want to say, "I'm not comfortable when you do that," or "I'm not ready for that." Then explain what you *do* want.

Above all, don't keep your likes and dislikes hidden from your partner, or you'll simmer with resentment when he or she fails to please you. Don't let the "bedroom misunderstanding syndrome" spoil your relationship. If you're uncomfortable talking about sexual matters, it is probably only because you haven't done much of it before.

The greatest sexual satisfaction in a relationship happens when both partners are able to be open and honest about what they like the most and what they like the least. There is always a certain amount of experimentation necessary to discover the fullest enjoyment of one's own body and the other person's body. You will like some things and not like others, but you will never know unless you and your partner experiment. It is always best to talk about your sex life with your partner. You'll be glad as you see your relationship growing stronger, deeper, and more satisfying for both of you.

The love-talk doesn't need to be a nonstop monologue the whole time. Keep it natural. Speak when you have something to say and only then. Make an effort to be pleasing in your tone of voice as well as in what you say.

In today's language, this would be called "extended foreplay," and it should, of course, lead to a fullness of sexual union. The difference is the talking and, after union, the slow, graceful movements aimed at enhancing and celebrating intimacy rather than driving for climax. The rhythm of this union should be more like the rhythm of a Vienna waltz than that of churning butter. At this time, one of the partners (the man, in Karezza) is to pour out his soul in as poetic expression of love as he can, letting it pour out like a slow-moving river.

Don't worry about awkwardness. Innocent, spontaneous expression with some awkwardness is far more real than smooth, over-practical "professionalism." For the man, there is a practical side to this vocal outpouring. Experts have found that verbal expression of the sounds of pleasure helps the man control and delay the time of climax.

The Karezza way doesn't require climax by either man or woman, since it emphasizes intimacy, harmony, and unity. It also takes a lot of practice to make it work right, and the couple wishing to practice Karezza should be patient. It takes time to harmonize energy fields, emotions, rhythms, and responses between two persons. Expect to practice at least a dozen times before you begin to see increasingly delightful results. The primary difficulty to overcome is the problem of control with the man.

THE WOMAN'S ROLE IN KAREZZA

In the original description of Karezza, the woman's role is more or less passive, although vital to its success. Rather than "passive," "cooperative" is a better term. We will discuss variations later, but first let's go over the original method.

The woman lies on her back next to the man, very still and as relaxed as possible. It is said that the cooperation of the woman can help turn the clumsiest man into a true lover, a poet of lovers. On the other hand, a woman who insists on passionate, thrusting, body movements will prevent the Karezza way from working, stimulating the man too quickly to climax.

Most men must learn to exercise control over the time of sexual climax, and Karezza is said to be the ideal way to assume that both partners are satisfied. If the woman is patient, she may reach heights of ecstasy unavailable through other methods of making love.

The original proponents of Karezza apparently tried reversing roles, having the woman be the active partner and the man be the passive partner. It didn't work. Whether the reasons were cultural or not remain to be seen. If a man doesn't feel threatened, fearful, or guilty over the woman's taking the active role, this variation of Karezza should work fine.

However, it may be that natural energy polarities make the pure form of Karezza work best when the man plays the active role and the woman the more passive role. Here the woman's passion must follow the man's, at least until the basic form of Karezza has been mastered.

The woman's role is to fantasize the man as her hero, one she greatly admires. The man is to see the woman as a person he cherishes, takes care of, protects. This attitude on the part of the woman appears critical to generating the energy interaction that can lift her to heights of ecstasy. Karezza is *not* designed as a manipulative, chauvinistic trick, but as a means of enhancing the natural femininity that precisely complements the natural masculinity of the man. This results in a balancing of sexual polarities.

If the woman holds to this expression of herself in Karezza, both partners become gradually lifted to a level of great passion, power, and security where any desired movements by either partner can be expressed, provided that they are expected by the other person and consistent with the rhythm of previous movements. No movement, however, should be continued too long or repetitiously or it will generate a climax. Both partners are to avoid movements that are sudden, jerky, or surprising. Nervous wriggling and impatient thrusting are to be avoided.

When we compare ordinary sex with Karezza, we notice that ordinary sex often spends itself in exhaustion and can even be followed by depression. On the other hand, Karezza is followed by exhilaration, a sense of power, and great satisfaction. It is heavenly music brought to earth. In Karezza, the aim is luxurious emotion, the beauty of relationships, sensual excitement, the subtlety of interaction, the gracefulness of dancing, the delight of pleasurable rhythm, and an appreciation that lingers.

THE SPIRITUAL ELEMENT OF KAREZZA

In this age of attitude conflicts between the sexes, it seems almost ironic that the ultimate and highest satisfaction for the woman lies so completely in her submission to the man. Similarly, it is ironic that the ultimate delight and satisfaction for the man, including his sense of triumph and pride, is so completely dependent on the woman.

Spiritually, however, the lesson is clear and makes a great deal of sense: To attain the most exalted state of happiness and fulfillment, it is necessary to help someone else get there, too. The intentions, cooperation, and actions of the woman make the difference between success and failure in Karezza. The man can cause failure, also, but he can't achieve success without the woman's cooperation. Neither can attain fullness of satisfaction without the complete, loving, harmonious help of the other.

What we should notice is that the spiritual principle of the Golden Rule is here: do unto others as you would have them do unto you. An even deeper principle is also evident. Only the one who serves can be lifted up; only the one who humbles himself can be exalted. Karezza teaches that we have to learn to put the other person first. When we do this in everyday relationships with others as well as in our love relationships, our lives will be transformed by following the spiritual principles.

HARMONY BETWEEN LOVE AND SEX

If we accept that life is first and foremost a spiritual realm of activity, we can see that misuse of our sexuality can lead to difficulty in relationships and to health problems. In fact, this is exactly what researchers are finding out in studies comparing sex-oriented relationships with love-oriented relationships. As I have said, we are all beings of body, mind, and spirit, not just body. Unless all three aspects of our humanity are working in harmony, life—and especially relationships—will never seem to be right. We have to pay attention to mind and spirit as well as to our bodies, or we will always sense something important missing in our lives.

Previously I have mentioned that the electromagnetic field around a woman is like that of the moon, a negative or attracting force. Similarly, the field around a man is like that of the sun, a positive or responding force. The two are opposites, and, of course, opposites attract. But unless opposites are in balance, in harmony, the result can be destructive, as is the case when one energy overpowers the other. In love relationships, our partnerships must be balanced in terms of the energy we radiate as well as in behavior, feelings, and attitudes.

Often I have said, "We are instruments of a million strings," referring to the many nerves in the body, over which high frequency, electromagnetic "melody-messages" are played. This is the music of life itself, more wonderful than we dare to imagine. This is the music of love.

Part Three
NUTRITION

Chapter Thirteen
Our Modern
"Disease"

Many people have asked me, "Do you understand why there are so many sex-related problems these days?" I always tell them, "Yes and no." It's a tough question to answer, because we live in tough times: confused times, unusual times.

It is ironic that sex problems are epidemic at a time when sexual freedom has never been greater. Just when we can do about anything we want to do, some have become sexual "gluttons," while others are frightened or intimidated by sex. We have women-hating men and men-hating women. We read about child abuse, parent abuse, and spouse abuse. The list of sexually-trans-mitted diseases (and the people who have had one or more) grows longer each year. AIDS, a deadly epidemic generated by sexual promiscuity, has arrived. The statistics on abortion compete with statistics on sterility. Terms like "fetal alcohol syndrome" and "fetal drug syndrome" are seen daily in news articles. And we've only begun to scratch the surface of solving these problems.

DIET AFFECTS SEX

Degeneration of the social and behavioral aspects of human sexu-ality are caused by many factors, but nutrition is unquestionably one of the foremost. Human sexuality is determined more by what we eat and how we live and work than by anything else. Most of our problems in human sexuality are coming from die-tary- and lifestyle burnout. We need to face these facts and make changes accordingly.

Along with their patients, doctors must begin to address the link between nutrition and health. It is not standard practice among most health professionals to look into a person's nutrition, exercise, and lifestyle to determine the cause of a health problem. Most doctors treat symptoms of disease, neglecting the basic cause of the problem and thereby virtually guarantee that new symptoms will reappear until the cause is dealt with directly.

As a clinical nutritionist, my goal has been correction of primary health problems rather than suppression of secondary symptoms. If we focus on suppressing symptoms alone, we are asking for a greater problem later, possibly greater than we can handle.

In all degenerative diseases, there is a point of no return, a moment when the person has "bought his ticket to the other side." I do not feel we have reached this point in our problems with sex; but we must realize that this nation could become both bankrupt and completely demoralized if we do not act to reverse the present mores of sexuality in our society.

To correct this problem, civilization must begin again. We must reevaluate the viability of our diets, our thinking, our morality. Our goal is to achieve a wonderful sex life for all by cleansing our bodies and minds of the old life and building a new, better, and cleaner life in its place.

ARE WE BECOMING A SEEDLESS SOCIETY?

Seeds are of great value to the human race because they are the glands of plants. They are whole, pure, natural foods containing everything necessary to build new life. When we eat seeds, we are taking vital glandular materials into our bodies and building up the integrity of our own glands and reproductive systems.

Unfortunately, when we eat white flour, white rice, and refined (dead) grain (seed) products, the life factors have been removed. As a result, these products no longer build the glands or protect the integrity of human fertility. And the great majority of people in our society are living solely on these refined, lifeless foods.

In many Western countries, we have developed a "seedless generation," a generation of men and women who lack vitality and integrity in their glands and hormones. Because the brain and glands interact, the sex center is also affected. As a result, the quality and expression of life has changed.

Child molestation, pornography, rape, abortion, violence between sex partners, bestiality, and homosexuality are common these days. I believe that the people responsible for these actions are the "seedless people," those whose bodies were unintentionally altered through degeneration in the quality of their food.

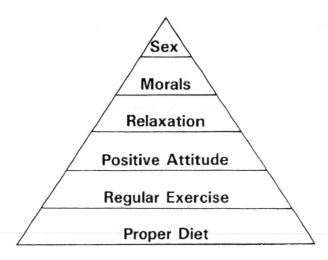

Foundations of a Super Sex Life

Everyone is hungry for normal sex. But when the body chemistry and glands are abnormal, the sexual expression is abnormal. Millions of people in the United States and other countries are deficient in their mental sex centers because they are deficient in the seed-derived, vital, gland-building materials once found in whole foods. Not only their glands, but also their minds and spirits, are affected.

CIVILIZATION OR DEGENERATION

Do we mold civilization, or does civilization mold us? The great inventions of one age seem to bring disaster in the next. The flour mills, the bleaching plants, and the chemical preservatives that once represented triumphs of food technology have created today's nutritional deficiencies.

Observe history. As our foods departed more and more from the whole, pure, and natural, the rise in chronic and degenerative diseases became epidemic. Was the "Sexual Revolution" of the 1960s a social revolution or merely another manifestation of the glandular degeneration and moral decline of Western civilization? We now have more disease, crime, and sex-related problems than ever before in the history of man.

The technological revolution has given us computers, color televisions, robotics, access to outer space, and a host of other wonderful advantages. But it has also made us a "sit-to" culture: "sit-to-work," "sit-to-drive," "sit-to-be-entertained." Likewise, technology's strides in food production have cheated us of valuable nutrients. Technology has perfected ways of processing, preserving, packaging, and mass-marketing foods. But these foods are devitalized because they are harvested from chemically-fertilized soils. Nutrient-deficient, inferior foods build health-deficient, inferior bodies and brains. Consequently, sickness and disease run rampant in Western bodies, minds, and behavior.

Because of these things, we need to take a hard look at how our civilization has degenerated and determine to take the higher path to a better way of life. We can reverse this state of affairs if we're willing to work and make changes.

THE SYMPTOMS OF OUR "DISEASE"

Every "symptom" exists in an environment of contributing causes, problems, mental attitudes, emotions, and thoughts. We have to treat the whole person on the other end of the symptom rather than the symptom itself or we will simply create more symptoms.

When a woman loses interest in sex, we recognize that the loss of interest is a mental thing. Yet, the problem is not in the mind alone. There is also a chemical side of the problem; a question of nutritional deficiencies, poor elimination; and possibly other ailments or diseases contributing to the problem.

If a man is incapable of having an erection, we know this is a physical problem. But the problem is not in the body alone. We must look into the realm of feelings, worries, anxieties, stress, and consider the possibility of depression as causes.

Likewise, we must search for underlying symptoms in our modern society that contribute to our modern disease.

Fear

Fear is a symptom of our modern disease.

Fear plays a part in absence of sexual desire, infertility, jealousy, rape, child molestation, sexually-transmitted diseases, and just about anything else that is not "working right" in sex. The greatest single source of fear in this history of man is war and the threat of war. At present, our children fear a nuclear war. Not long ago, a generation of young Americans fought in the Vietnam War. Virtually every human being now alive is able to recall a time when war was raging during their lives.

War

War is a symptom of our modern disease.

The Vietnam war was the most socially-destructive event of our century, despite such anti-war slogans as "Make Love, Not War."

War creates an aura of adventurous glamour which tolerates social behavior that is considered unacceptable in peacetime. Wives left at home commit adultery. Husbands in the military visit prostitutes, and sometimes even rape civilians. Drug- and alcohol-abuse increase.

War accelerates chemical pollution and destruction of the land. Agent Orange, the defoliant used in Vietnam, not only ravaged natural vegetation, but also destroyed the sex lives of soldiers and civilians who were exposed to it.

The presence of death and dying cheapens the value of all human life not just during the war, but for years after. Postwar periods are full of increased crime, violence, and disregard for law and morals as citizens readjust to the discipline of peacetime morality.

Stress

Stress is a symptom of our modern disease.

A "cousin" of fear, stress also contributes to loose morality as people "unwind" from job pressures, freeway driving, financial problems, and the noise and confusion of daily events.

Stress can cause nerve acids to build up faster than they are eliminated, leading to cell damage in inherently weak organs, glands, and tissues. Stress can cause constipation, resulting in increased levels of toxic material in the bloodstream. The adrenal glands, important to healthy sexual function, can be depleted by stress, as can the thyroid gland, often called the "emotion gland."

The studies of Dr. Hans Selye showed that stress can bring damage to almost any organ or body system. Two of the first symptoms of stress are often increasingly chronic fatigue and increasingly frequent depression. Along with this unfortunate pair of symptoms—one a result of stress on the body, the other a result

of stress on the mind—nearly always comes loss of sexual desire
or interest. When we are depressed, the immune system does not
work as well. Making love might increase the endorphine output
in the brain and raise the immune level—if only fatigue and depression did not sabotage our efforts to make love at all.

Drugs

Drug abuse is a symptom of our modern disease.

Some say that alcohol and drugs such as marijuana and cocaine
are aphrodisiacs, that is, substances purported to increase sexual
desire. They can lower the level of inhibition (especially alcohol),
while reducing the ability to respond and participate. Marijuana
creates the illusion of prolonging sex and sometimes intensifying
pleasurable feelings over the short term, but reduces sexual enjoyment and interest over the long term. (The exact time varies with
the individual.) With cocaine, sex is amplified to a larger-than-life
pleasure; but soon, it is the cocaine that becomes the center of
desire, not the lover or the lovemaking. For this, and other reasons, cocaine is both addictive and dangerous.

Most doctors agree by now that the so-called "pleasure drugs"
wipe out interest in sex sooner or later. In this sense, they are
actually sexual depressants or repressants, not sexual stimulants. I
have spoken with many people who have given up drugs and
alcohol to take a higher path to health and life. They tell me that
nothing in their "drug-use" days compares with sex at the peak of
well-being. They say that good health is a greater source of joy
than drugs can ever be.

Generally speaking, addictions of any kind reduce the enjoyment of sex. There can be many reasons for this. One is that
addictions reduce the health level and the quality of relationships
at the same time. There is an erosion of the capacity to enjoy sex,
on the one hand, and a loss of interest in the person one with
whom one has sex, on the other hand.

People talk about "getting high." I believe the best way to "get
high" is to take a higher path in life, to learn to make each
moment more satisfying, more focused, more enjoyable for others
as well as oneself.

Sometimes I feel that man's interest in sexual stimulants is a
result of pure laziness, another means of trying to avoid the work
of developing intimate relationships. Let's face it, good relationships require hard work. But, as with much of life's other efforts,

the hard work pays off. The intimacy of a loving relationship always provides the greatest sex we can experience.

So, in conclusion, let's pledge to be more aware of this disease that is permeating our society as well as the effects of all its symptoms. We have to really understand the disease before we can hope to find the cure. It is only then that we can work to establish truly satisfactory loving and sexual relationships.

Chapter Fourteen
The Four Stages of Disease

All of us have inherent strengths and weaknesses that come as part of our genetic inheritance. We hear doctors say, "He has weak kidneys," or "She has a weak digestive system." Inherent strengths are genetically-inherited strong and healthy organs, glands, and tissues that seldom give us any problem. It is the weakest link in a chain that breaks first, and like the weak links in a chain, it is the inherently weak organs, glands, tissues, and brain centers that must be cared for the most.

Inherently weak brain centers can become weakened and deficient in minerals by overwork. Any overworked brain center requires abnormal expenditures of energy to operate and is subject to toxic deposits—but not the same toxic deposits as we find in the body. Because of the blood/brain barrier, chemical access to the brain is restricted for protective reasons. However, it isn't restrictive enough. Alcohol, Valium, and many other harmful substances can get past it.

Inherently weak tissues assimilate nutrients and expel wastes more slowly than normal tissues. They seem to function at a slower metabolic rate. Because of this, they need a slight overabundance of vitamins, minerals, and other important nutrients to function normally and to remain free of disease and dysfunction. When we don't take care of ourselves, it is the inherent weaknesses that suffer from inflammation, underactivity, and toxic accumulations. Drug residues or catarrh settle in these tissues, where they become irritants and sources of inflammation.

Inherent weaknesses in the sexual system may be found in the primary sex system—hypothalamus of the brain (sex center), cerebellum (sex drive), endocrine glands (sex hormones), and nervous system (sensory, motor and autonomic nerves related to sexual function).

However, the sexual system, even if it were inherently strong, could be affected by secondary body systems such as the digestive system, the elimination system, the circulatory system, and various organs, glands, and tissues (such as the liver, pancreas, and skin) which could dramatically interfere with the sex life.

If your heart is inherently weak and underactive, for example, it doesn't matter how wildly romantic and sexual your mental centers are, you are going to have to be somewhat careful about your sexual expression.

Similarly, if the testes of a man are inherently weak and his male hormone production is low, his sex drive will be physically weak even though his sexual desire (mental) may be quite strong.

THE FOUR STAGES OF DISEASE

All diseases progress through four stages: acute, subacute, chronic, and degenerative, spanning a time period ranging from a few months to a lifetime. (See following chart.) Diseases don't occur by accident. We work for them. We earn them. We have to eat, drink, and think them into existence.

Every disease begins with the acute, "overactive" stage, in which irritation or injury produces inflammation in some specific tissue area. Inflammation brings on increased blood supply, hormonal secretions to bring down swelling, increased lymph, and greater nerve activity. If metabolic overactivity doesn't get rid of the problem, the tissue goes to the subacute stage.

When the initial warning of acute symptoms is ignored or suppressed, the original cause (and the catarrh produced in response to it) are driven into the tissue and remain there. The metabolic response of the tissue shifts from overactivity to underactivity. Symptoms may disappear. (Even some acute reactions may be undetectable by lab tests or physical exam.)

With time, toxic accumulations in the underactive, subacute tissue increase in quantity and effect, further reducing the functional level. Symptoms may appear at this stage simply because the functional level of the tissue is so low that the identifying characteristics of a disease emerge. This is the chronic stage.

The degenerative stage is such an extreme state of underactivity that the disease may be irreversible.

Keep in mind that autonomic nerve messages are keeping the

The Four Stages of Disease

Acute: Fevers, development of phlegm, catarrh and mucus, discharges, all "itises" (the class of inflammations that include tonsillitis, sinusitis, gastritis, vaginitis, and bronchitis) and extreme acidity.

Subacute: Poor circulation, joint pains, continuous aches, constipation, fatigue, lack of stomach hydrochloric acid, slower metabolism, hypocalcemia, and depletion of will and morale.

Chronic: Poor assimilation, poor oxygenation, inherent weaknesses beginning to break down, poor function in inherently weak organs, extreme chemical deficiencies, rheumatism, symptoms subside, bowel transit time increases, exhaustion, vital energies low, damaged tissue not being repaired, immune system breakdown, suppressed catarrh no longer runs, faulty mental concentration.

Degenerative: All four elimination channels underactive, complete breakdown of inherent weaknesses, maximum toxic settlements, complete vital organ breakdown, complete symptom suppression, complete breakdown of vital force, arthritis, osteoporosis, joint deformities, mental functions and alertness diminish.

brain informed (particularly the hypothalamus, a major nerve relay in the brain) of what is going on in the tissue.

Normally, the lymph and blood carry immune system cells to the afflicted area, and these cells try to remove accumulated toxic materials. Often, they can't do it, because the lymph system and the elimination channels have become overburdened and underactive during the developmental stages of the disease.

When the elimination channels—the bowel, kidneys, skin, lungs, and bronchial tubes—become underactive, the toxic levels in the blood and lymph are even higher, creating a very dangerous condition for all inherently weak tissues in the body.

Let's follow the course of two diseases, atherosclerosis and emphysema, to illustrate the pathway to disease I am describing here. I'll then relate this illustration to sexual dysfunction.

The Acute Stage

The lifestyle here may vary from childhood to a young adult's simple, pleasure-seeking lifestyle or that of the hard-working career person. Many meals are rushed or carelessly put together, resulting in inadequate fiber, fruit, vegetables, and a generally imbalanced diet, containing too much fried, fatty foods, too much sugar, too much wheat and milk in the diet. Staying up too late or working too hard increases fatigue acids in the body. Smoking, drinking alcoholic beverages, using drugs (including diet pills)—lowers the efficiency of the lungs, liver, and brain, and interferes with blood circulation and fat metabolism. Children may be seriously affected by the cigarette smoke of adults around them. Other factors contributing to acute diseases may be involved, such as exposure to X-rays, ultraviolet radiation, air pollution, food and drinking water with chemical additives, pesticide sprays, sexual abuse, emotional or physical abuse, and a history of disease in the family.

Inside the body, chemicals or microorganisms may be attacking the linings of blood vessels, particularly the interfaces between cells that form the linings of blood vessels. No one really knows the causes of atherosclerosis, but the initial phases of the disease have been clearly observed. In response to cell-boundary inflammation, calcium plaque begins to form over the damaged areas. This is the very beginning of atherosclerosis. In the nasal passages, sinuses, bronchials, and lungs, irritation from airborne pollutants, cigarette smoke, dust, plant pollen, perfumes, household- or industrial chemical vapors causes inflammations.

In the external environment, arguments between parents (or with parents), emotional ups and downs, job stress, problems with the boyfriend, girlfriend, or spouse, feelings of inadequacy, being unjustly treated or being ignored—all these and other mental and spiritual problems add up to alter the endocrine gland functions, brain center functions, nerve functions, acid/alkaline balance of the body, and (often) bowel regularity. These emotional ups and downs contribute to acidity in the body which aggravates any inflammation. A spastic or constipated bowel increases the amount of toxic materials in the bloodstream, which further irritate the tissues, delay healing, and stimulate more catarrh.

Although there are no acute symptoms of atherosclerosis, the presence of frequent colds, fevers, coughs, bronchial irritation, allergies, and flu signal the kind of lung weakness that can lead in the long run to asthma and emphysema.

The Subacute Stage

The usual response to catarrhal discharges and conditions like colds, coughs, and fevers is to use suppressant drugs. This drives catarrh back into the tissues and suppresses the overactive tissue function so it becomes underactive. The tissue inflammation remains, but now it is present in a context of metabolic weakness and underactivity.

While in the subacute stage, tissues may not show symptoms, but toxic materials are slowly being accumulated nonetheless. In blood vessels, greasy smears of cholesterol and fats are found to be clinging to the rough calcium-coated scars along the borders of cells in the blood vessel lining. In the lungs and bronchials, toxic deposits and progressive underactivity go hand in hand. Dried catarrh, chemical pollutants, and suppressant drug residues are imbedded in the tissues. Carbon dioxide is not eliminated as rapidly as it should be, and oxygen intake is below normal. This increases the acidity of the body and lowers brain efficiency.

In terms of health level, the subacute stage is not a real problem time for those developing atherosclerosis or chronic/degenerative lung conditions. Life is pleasant, and no physical limitations are yet apparent, because the physical changes take place so slowly. Episodes of colds, flus, sinusitis, hay fever, and bronchitis may come and go, but usually not enough to discourage habits like cigarette smoking, excess alcohol, drug abuse, or workaholism.

Neither men nor women would normally notice any change in their sex lives at either the acute or subacute stages of disease development.

I want to point out that diet is a critical factor in the progression of atherosclerosis. A high-fat diet accelerates this disease. Countries in which the per capita consumption of beef and dairy products is highest also have the highest rates of cardiovascular disease.

The Chronic Stage

At the chronic stage of disease, problems of a variety of kinds begin to be evident. Internally, a decrease of blood, lymph, and innervation to the affected tissue is evident. Nutrients are scarcely able to get into the tissues, and metabolic wastes can hardly get out. Toxic substances in the blood, at this point, are being transferred to inherently weak tissues other than the primary problem area of the body.

The onset of fatigue is evident at this point, which may have a mild-to-devastating effect on the sex life. A great deal of available energy is being used to detoxify the area around the lungs in one case, and reduced blood flow and lower oxygenation is producing a similar low-energy problem with atherosclerosis. Symptoms may include obesity, high blood pressure, sensations of heaviness in the chest, and easy cramping of the muscles. Diabetes (high blood sugar) and depression are frequently associated with atherosclerosis, and both of these may interfere with the sex life.

There are three specific sex-related problems associated with chronic atherosclerosis. One is the combined effects of low energy/mental depression, which reduces desire. The second is the blockage of blood flow to the groin, which hinders arousal in both men and women. The third is the effect of medications for high blood pressure or for depression, either of which may affect both libido and sexual ability. Mood-changing drugs and blood pressure drugs are well-known for their negative effects on the sex life.

Symptoms of chronic asthma/emphysema include periodic disabling attacks of coughing, wheezing, upper respiratory infections, difficulty breathing, physical weakness, insomnia, restlessness, and general physical discomfort. During these attacks, sex is generally out of the question. Between attacks of asthma or emphysema, an active sex life can be maintained, but with a lower level of energy and frequent breathing difficulties.

The Degenerative Stage

All through the first three stages of disease—acute, subacute, and chronic—the body copes and compensates for the progressive changes of the disease. At the degenerative stage, this compensation begins to lose ground.

Internally, the tissue has reached a stage of total or nearly total inactivity. In atherosclerosis, this means that arteries are almost completely choked with fatty deposits. When the arteries of the heart are radically blocked, bypass surgery may be performed. Impotence due to blocked groin arteries can be reversed by surgery, but at the degenerative stage it may be questionable whether a person is still interested in sex.

I don't like to say that the degenerative stage is the end of the road. It may not be for some courageous persons. But for many, a degenerative disease in one part of the body means there are serious problems in other parts of the body as well, problems brought on by the lifestyle that brought on the degenerative disease.

In emphysema, for example, the tiny air sacs of the lungs are broken down, and there is no way to repair them. It is possible to slow down progress of the disease but not to stop it. Oxygen intake is reduced, which hampers brain efficiency and heart function, and carbon dioxide is not being expelled as rapidly as it should be. Internal stress from "air hunger" usually leads to adrenal-gland exhaustion. Energy reserves are depleted. The four elimination channels (bowel, kidneys, skin, lungs, and bronchials) are underactive, and a high level of toxins circulate in the blood and lymph, creating serious problems for all inherent weaknesses in the body.

By the time any disease has reached the degenerative stage, stress from the presence of the disease is affecting the endocrine gland system and the brain centers. This is complicated by high levels of toxic materials in the blood and lymph brought on by underactive elimination channels. The nerves are irritated by the overacid condition in the body, also due to stress and high levels of toxins.

Where is sex in all this? Usually gone. In fact, it is being slowly undermined as any disease develops in the body. The sex life is eroded by diminishing energy resources, increasing acidity in the body, irritated nerves, increasing levels of toxins in the blood and lymph, endocrine depletion and imbalance, fatigue, and a lowering of function in brain centers. This occurs whether or not there is any inherent weakness in the sexual system. The only difference is that it happens much faster when the sexual system is inherently weak.

SEX SYMPTOMS—ONE APPROACH

All sex symptoms must be taken care of in the overall context of your life—what environment you are in and what your life feels like to you on the inside. You are capable of changing both the external environment and the internal environment. It is my sincere belief that it is mistaken and ineffective to treat only symptoms by giving a patient a Band-Aid, a pill, or a little advice to take care of the symptom. At the end of any symptom is the other 99 percent of the person. That's what we must focus on keeping healthy.

If you lack interest in sex, you probably are not enjoying the rest of your life all that well, either. In the process of dealing with the larger problem—the smaller one will be solved.

If you are not feeling much pleasure in sex, perhaps your circulation or innervation is not what it should be. Maybe it is not a psychological problem at all. Try building up your circulation by exercise and nutrition before going to a doctor or psychological counselor. Give your nerves more rest and use high lecithin foods or supplements.

Don't try to treat symptoms—look for the causes of the symptoms and take care of them. As we will see in the next chapter, the holistic approach to taking care of people involves the body, mind, and spirit. You are inseparably all three. For this reason, you must not neglect any one aspect of your being.

On the physical level, this means you must always be conscious of your overall diet—what you eat three times daily—as well as the amount of regular exercise you get, and your bad habits, before you resort to visiting a doctor to determine the cause of your maladies.

On the spiritual and psychological levels, there are principles involved to breaking out of the kinds of ruts that create problems, as well. First, be good to yourself—don't wait around for someone to come up and be good to you. Second, love others—for your own good, whether or not they love you in return. Avoid negative people at all times. Be around people who love you. Learn to forgive and forget. Remember, what you put your attention to, grows. So always have your attention on some wonderful thought or goal.

Chapter Fifteen

The Holistic Treatment

Just as we learned about the *existence* of a four-stage pattern for the development of a chronic or degenerative disease, we must also learn about the *nature* of that pattern to understand more about love, sex, and nutrition.

Nature's way of healing (as contrasted with drug treatment or surgery) involves a reversal of the four-stage pathway to disease. The holistic health perspective, which is based on this philosophy, teaches that man is made of three levels: body, mind, and spirit. Sexual problems or health problems of any kind can be caused at any of these three levels.

Spiritual problems that result in guilt or shame, mental troubles like worry, or physical processes such as not eating right and not getting enough sleep, can disrupt a person's sex life. Moreover, whether a problem begins in the spirit, mind, or body, it always affects the other two levels, and—sooner or later—it will show up in the body.

HERING'S LAW OF CURE

Nineteenth-century European homeopath Constantine Hering discovered the law that governs all natural healing: "All cure comes from the inside out, from the head down, and in reverse order as the symptoms first appeared."

A nutshell explanation of Hering's Law is that cure begins inside the body as the causes of the problem are removed. This process comes "from the head down" in the sense that the brain directs and correlates all healing processes. As healing commences, the most recent internal tissue damage is corrected first, while the original symptoms and manifestations are taken care of last, *in reverse order as symptoms first appeared.*

Hering's Law describes the reversal process that characterizes all natural forms of healing. Non-natural forms of healing use either treatment with drugs, which suppress symptoms and alter the internal chemistry of the body, or treatment with surgery, which often involves the removal of part of the body. There is no tissue correction in either surgery or treatment with drugs. Tissue correction happens only through natural healing methods in which damaged tissue is rebuilt and replaced.

In other words, the natural healing methods that I have taught for over fifty-five years bring about a reversal of the path of disease—in the direction of improved health. If the sex drive has been lost, it will be recovered again at the same point on the reversal pathway where it was first lost. Glandular balance may be similarly restored and the full enjoyment of sex that was once there.

A healing crisis is the body's natural reaction when the healing power of the body displaces the conditions of disease. Its tendency is toward recovery. A healing crisis is the result of a quickened effort by every organ and tissue in the body to throw off toxic settlements and set the stage for replacing the old tissue with new tissue.

Just as a pathway to disease can be discovered that shows the gradual development of disease through the acute, subacute, chronic, and degenerative stages, the pathway to health is found in backtracking along the pathway to disease.

The reversal process retraces the steps of a disease by substituting steps toward health. Beginning the reversal process may entail dropping habits that are contributing to or favoring the disease process, changing one's food regimen, getting regular exercise and rest, and adopting positive attitudes in place of negative attitudes.

Before we can build up the body and sex life, we have to stop what is breaking it down. This requires an honest self-appraisal and the resolve to replace destructive habits with constructive ones.

A habit is a behavior that tends to be compulsive or that we repeat frequently without conscious thought. Excessive drinking, cigarette smoking, and using drugs like cocaine, heroin, Valium, and amphetamines are only the tip of the habit "iceberg." How about food habits—fried foods, wheat products, salty foods, milk products, sugar, chocolate, sweet desserts, commercial soft drinks, coffee, tea, and others? How about thought habits—hate, bitterness, vengefulness, jealousy, shame, guilt, fear, resentment, and rebellion? What about behavioral habits—not sleeping enough, seldom exercising, complaining, working too hard? These are habits that can contribute to diseases by causing us to break down faster than we can build up.

When we have stopped breaking down the body, we need to pay attention to taking care of our nervous systems and our eliminative organs. We need to cleanse the body of toxins and build up its strength. Our blood and lymph will not be free of toxic material until our elimination channels are cleaned and restored.

Often, the process of healing can be accelerated with the seven-day cleansing program, described in my book *Tissue Cleansing Through Bowel Management*. There are also various kinds of fasts that can increase the rate of tissue cleansing. Fasting, though, *should always be done under the supervision of a doctor or nutritionist.*

You will never realize how accumulated catarrh, wastes, and toxins in the tissues can drag down your energy and vitality until you experience being free from them. Fasting should not be regarded as unpleasant or difficult but as an enjoyable process of restoration, of "lightening-up," of getting on top of things again. Getting rid of toxic buildup is a necessary part of the reversal process, and although we can partly rid ourselves of toxins by fasting, it is necessary to go further; to go through the healing crisis to bring about elimination of the most deeply-imbedded toxins.

A balanced food regimen is absolutely necessary to follow the reversal path to good health. I'll get into that in detail later, but first I want to point out that only food can build new tissue. Drugs are sometimes necessary and useful, but they cannot build new tissue. There is no therapy in the healing art that will assist in bringing about healing without nutrition to help it. And, further, there is no therapy that won't progress much more rapidly when a balanced, effective food regimen is used with it. Therefore, only food can bring tissue correction.

Although I respect the vegetarian way very much, you can't rebuild a broken-down sex system or enhance a normal one on vegetables alone. There is a need for animal proteins and fats, the more highly-evolved foods, to build up the sex system. Vegetarianism favors celibacy, and that is not what this book is about.

There are seven priorities we need to have in taking care of the body.

1. We need to be aware of, and take care of, our inherent weaknesses, keeping the body clean and well-fed.
2. Toxic accumulations will develop in any inherently weak tissue that is deficient in the necessary chemical elements.
3. The chemical elements (see Chapter Seventeen) needed by the body must be provided by the food we eat. Every disease is characterized by specific nutritional deficiencies. To avoid disease, we must have a balanced food regimen.
4. The blood must be clean (free of toxic material) and must include the proper balance of nutrients.
5. Circulation of the blood is just as important as what the blood contains. Exercise (see Chapter Twenty-Three) is required for proper circulation.
6. Elimination channels—the bowel, kidneys, skin, lungs, and bronchials—must be kept clean to avoid toxins getting into the bloodstream.
7. Innervation—getting adequate nerve communication to all organs, glands, and tissues of the body—is essential to our well-being.

The heart and all other muscles are favored by potassium foods. The digestive and eliminative systems are favored by sodium foods. The brain, nerves, glands, and sexual system are favored by foods high in phosphates, silicon, fatty acids, and zinc. We need to replenish chemical elements by eating a variety of whole, pure, and natural foods.

To bring about a healing crisis, our strategy is to strengthen not just the part of the body affected by disease but the whole body. This is because the whole body participates in the casting off of disease—and so does the mind.

Psychosomatic diseases, such as ulcers, are created by our thoughts and emotions, but the truth is, every disease has a psychosomatic component. Nerve relays from the cortex, the limbic system, and every organ, gland, and tissue in the body meet in the hypothalamus of the brain. Every thought and emotion we have interacts with every cell in our bodies. Depression suppresses our immune system activity. Love and affection increase it. Hate and unforgiveness contribute to cancer, heart disease, and arthritis. Forgiveness is part of the healing process. Guilt and shame may contribute to a disease and can be imbedded so deeply that only spiritual counselling can get it out.

To trigger a healing crisis in the body, we want to bring our bodies, minds, and spirits to the highest degree of health and strength possible, while removing as many obstacles to reversal as possible by breaking up old habits and cleaning up our "mental act."

FROM THE INSIDE OUT

As we increase the health and strength of our bodies through proper eating, exercise, and rest, the condition of our internal organs, glands, and tissues begins to backtrack to the first stage of active manifestation of disease. The symptoms appear once again—fever, headaches, running nose, lung congestion—and catarrhal elimination may take place through any or all orifices of the body. In cases such as atherosclerosis, there are no obvious physical manifestations of disease, but there is a reversal and cleansing nonetheless.

Nathan Pritikin, the man who developed the Pritikin Diet for those with cardiovascular disease, died in his sixties. He once had advanced atherosclerosis, but because he stuck to a low-fat diet and high-exercise regimen, he was able to reverse the disease. An autopsy at his death showed that his arteries were as clean as those of a teenage boy. (Pritikin died of leukemia.)

I believe that atherosclerosis, along with other diseases, can be reversed with proper diet and exercise.

As we adopt new eating habits and better lifestyles, our bodies mold to the new pattern. New tissue replaces the old tissue. Our level of health retraces backward along the same route that led us into the disease in the first place. We may experience a series of healing crises that repeat the symptoms of past stages of the disease we are working to eliminate—including some of the emotional and mental symptoms. Each crisis comes at a point where the replacement of new tissue is ready and able to throw off more of the old catarrh and tissue-bound toxic material.

THE HEALING CRISIS

A healing crisis can't be forced and doesn't always come after a period of fasting or bowel cleansing. It comes when it is ready, when all organs, glands, and tissues are ready to add their support. If the mind is not ready (holding onto some deep worry or regret) the crisis may not take place.

The differences between a healing crisis and a disease crisis are primarily two-fold. First, a healing crisis usually comes suddenly at a time when we are feeling our best, while a disease crisis and its symptoms usually surface as part of a continuous downhill progression where a person feels worse and worse. Second, a healing crisis usually lasts three days or less, although I've known of some longer exceptions.

No two healing crises are alike, even with the same disease that causes them. Because everyone has lived differently, the reversal path to health will bring out different experiences and symptoms during the crises.

A person's appetite is generally low or absent during a healing crisis, and it is best to follow the body's lead. You should drink water to help carry off toxins and to replace water that has been lost, and rest as much as possible. If the person has been eating well up to the time of the healing crisis, there will be a reservoir or nutrients to last until the crisis is over. We must consider that disease is an abnormal state, and a healing crisis is part of the process of normalization.

It is unrealistic to expect that we can reverse ten, twenty, or fifty years of wrong living habits with a single, three-day healing crisis. Usually there is a series of crises—at least six months apart, depending on how rapidly new tissue is replacing the old. I advise my patients that they can't expect to be completely well in less than a year.

The symptoms of a healing crisis can be upsetting in their severity, but I have never known of a single person who couldn't get through one.

There can be diarrhea; gas; skin eruptions; rash; discharges from the ears, nose, vagina, and eyes; vomiting; coughing; fever; perspiration; pain anywhere in the body; emotional distress; and recollection of unpleasant memories or emotions as far back as childhood.

A word of caution: True healing is only accomplished through a healing crisis. Anyone in the health arts who knows what he or she is doing can temporarily stimulate overactivity in an organ or organ system. This will increase the absorption of nutrients and expulsion of wastes temporarily, but it won't have lasting results because overall correction has not been accomplished. Support from the other organs and glands of the body is necessary before a real healing crisis can take place. True healing requires a reorientation and reharmonizing of a formerly diseased organ or system with the whole community of organs and tissues.

FROM THE HEAD DOWN

It is a mental law that thought directs energy. Therefore, when we are reversing an inadequate or unsatisfactory sex life or even enhancing a good one, we need to be aware of what we are doing. I would rate our thinking as more important than the nutrients we take in, because our decisions not only determine our food habits, but also what we do with our lives.

"Outpicturing" through imagination is a powerfully effective way of helping (or hurting) the sex life. For example, an undisciplined imagination can be influenced, by pornography, toward a debased lifestyle. A disciplined imagination, on the other hand, can lead the way to such high-level well-being that morality is an integral and normal aspect of the way we consider sex enhancing our love lives while reinforcing the health of our minds.

To accelerate the reversal process, we organize our thoughts in support of what we are doing. Keep your mind on the goal— better health and a wonderful sex life. Love yourself, let go of the past, forgive and forget, and resolve that each tomorrow will be better than the last.

Chapter Sixteen
Sex and Nutrition

In the narrow sense, the sex problems we are looking at in this book include loss of sex drive, lack of sex interest (which may differ from the preceding), impotence, premature climax, sterility, damage to the pelvic organs (which may inhibit pleasure and encourage infections), inherent weaknesses in the sex system, diet- or lifestyle-related fatigue, and various other problems.

Psychological sex problems fall into a special category. But good diet and exercise are necessary even when counselling is the primary means of correction. Some problems may be primarily rooted in chemical or glandular imbalance and may be completely corrected by diet and exercise.

The distinction between psychological and spiritual problems is not always clear. The psychological consequences of rape, incest, molestation, or emotional intimidation often have a dimension that requires spiritual counselling from a priest, pastor, or rabbi. Not only the victims, but also the perpetrators, need competent corrective counsel.

SEX PROBLEMS PREY ON A MALNOURISHED BODY

Dr. William Albrecht, former head of the Department of Agriculture at the University of Missouri, once planted two identical seeds in two pots of soil—one containing mineral-rich topsoil, the other containing topsoil depleted in calcium and iron. The seeds sprouted and grew into vines, entwining with one another. The foliage of the one grown in rich soil was dark green and glossy, while the leaves of the other were pale, translucent, "anemic-looking."

As the two plants grew together, the sickly plant picked up viruses, bacterial colonies, and bugs. The fascinating thing was that none of them invaded the healthy plant, even though the two were so close.

When the food we eat lacks essential vitamins, minerals, enzymes, and other nutrients, we become undernourished and subject to disease. Food can become deficient in two ways: if grown in depleted soil, or if processed or cooked. For example, scurvy and beri-beri are two deficiency diseases that most doctors are familiar with; scurvy being caused by a lack of vitamin C, and beri-beri by a lack of thiamine, one of the B-vitamins.

Likewise, sexual problems, whether physical or mental, result from deficiencies—in knowledge, in attitude, in diet, in lifestyle. Once we correct the deficiency, the problem takes care of itself. This is Nature's way.

WE MUST FEED THE MIND

The mind has needs just as the body has needs. Love is one of the basic needs of the mind, but there are others, as well. All of us have known people who seem constantly in a stew of dissatisfaction. There is something missing in their lives. They sense the hunger, the lack, but they may not know what it is or how to remedy the situation. They are nervous, fidgety, frustrated. They may take up alcohol or drugs to alleviate the constant, nagging sense of incompleteness. They may be compulsive or impulsive in matters of love and sex.

We all need beauty, friendship, recreation, exposure to nature, challenge, meaningful work, a sense of self-worth, and other mental "foods." We all need some means of creative self-expression, such as art, drama, music, or a sport or hobby. That is, our minds have a need to receive, to take in, to appreciate and enjoy, but also our minds need to express, to give out, to perform, participate, or display.

Deficiencies in these mental "foods" can cause mental problems just as nutrient-deficiencies can cause physical problems. What complicates matters is that mental deficiencies can trigger physical problems, and nutrient deficiencies can also trigger mental problems! There is a close relationship between the mind and the body, each affecting the other. In fact, every thought and emotion affects every cell in the body, and everything that happens in and to the body affects the mind.

Sex may "exercise" the reproductive system, but unless love is present, the mind and heart are not fed. A husband may be handsome, rich, important in public life or business, and skilled in the methodology of sexual technique, but if he does not spend time showing his wife he loves and cares for her, she won't feel fulfilled in the relationship. Similarly, if the wife fears or dislikes sex for some reason, not only will her needs not be met; her husband will be frustrated, as well.

If we fail to feed our minds what is needed, something else will take its place. We could call this the law of compensation.

Many of us substitute routine activities for the mental and spiritual "food" we miss. Women may become pet-minded, children-minded, candy-minded, all of which are substitutes for the love they need. Men may become hobby-minded, sports-minded, or TV-minded. Think of all the women addicted to daytime soap operas, or all the men addicted to golf, bowling, or TV sports shows. This is the law of compensation at work. The real need is mental—love or some other form of fulfillment.

Boredom and marital conflict are often symptoms of mental starvation (or misunderstanding) without compensation taking place. However, it is only a matter of time before trouble comes in and fulfills the law of compensation. We all need to be noticed, to be appreciated, to be praised—and to be reprimanded or corrected if we are violating the rules of right relationship. Love includes these things. Of course, most people need to be told they are loved and need to be touched, hugged, and held frequently. Touching relationships nourish the mind as well as the body.

To paraphrase Dr. Albrecht's claim, "Sex problems prey on an undernourished mind as well as an undernourished body." We must feed both the mind and the body.

BODIES NEED TO BE WHOLE

Our bodies are made of food chemicals, and the energy we use is fueled by food chemicals. When some of these chemicals are lacking, certain parts of our bodies may be incomplete, so they cannot perform the functions they were designed to perform. Since we get the chemicals we need from foods, we have to have a variety of whole, pure, and natural foods to meet all the chemical needs of the body. We have to eat right, or our bodies will not work correctly.

Technically, as I have pointed out, our sex lives depend on the structural integrity of several glands, organs, and tissues of the body as well as on the availability of sufficient energy to perform at its best. Each of these parts of the sex system requires constant replenishing of the nutrients it requires. While the brain, nerves, and glands are fed by the same foods, different tissues require different foods to function at peak efficiency. Thus, a variety of nutrients needed by different tissues requires a variety of foods to supply those nutrients.

But suppose we were not getting the right foods to produce the sex hormones our bodies needed? We would be in serious trouble as far as our sex lives were concerned. Yet, it is not entirely what we eat that counts, but what we digest and assimilate, what we actually take into the bloodstream as nutrients ready for cells to use, that makes the difference.

The food we eat is primarily digested in the stomach and small intestine. In the stomach, hydrochloric acid breaks down proteins for further digestion in the small intestine. Biochemical sodium protects the stomach walls from being dissolved by hydrochloric acid, and sodium from the intestinal walls begins to neutralize acid-laden foods as they move from the stomach into the small intestine. There, pancreatic juices, bile from the gall bladder, and intestinal secretions complete the job of digestion.

Microscopic digested food particles in the small intestine are then assimilated through the intestinal wall by means of tiny, fingerlike projections called villi. The nutrients are picked up by the blood and lymphatic systems and transported first to the liver where proteins, carbohydrates, and fats are reformulated into nutrients ready for the various cells of the body to use. As these nutrients travel through the blood and lymph, different types of tissues draw on these nutrients to get the exact chemical combinations they need. The bones, for example, need calcium, phosphates, magnesium, and carbonate more than anything else.

If we aren't digesting and assimilating our foods properly, a balanced diet will become imbalanced by the time nutrients reach the blood and lymph. So if we aren't taking care of our stomachs and other digestive organs, we are promoting trouble for the whole body and for inherently weak organs, glands, and tissues, specifically.

When we eat, our highest priority must be to properly feed our digestive system. We need to have the right foods to keep our hydrochloric acid in balance with sodium in the stomach and small intestine. Many people have an imbalance between the acid and sodium. We need to have the right foods to keep the pancreatic and intestinal juices flowing, and enough fiber foods to get rid of excess bile and move wastes along at the proper rate. The digestive system needs leafy green vegetables as well as foods rich in sodium, such as whey, okra, celery, seafood, kelp, eggs, and cheese. (Table salt contains chemical sodium which is not natural.)

ONE OF MY MOST VALUABLE DISCOVERIES

Foods that often cause trouble in the digestive systems of many people include sugar, alcohol, milk, and wheat. As I have pointed out, studies have shown that the average American diet is 29 percent wheat products, 25 percent milk products, and 9 percent sugar. The gluten in wheat may clog the intestine, while milk irritates, and alcohol and sugar cause dehydration and fermentation in it. In my view, we should reduce milk and wheat products to 6 percent of the total dietary intake. We can get a better balance of nutrients from raw nuts, seeds, and grains such as brown rice, cornmeal, millet, buckwheat, and rye. In addition, most people over the age of 40 should be taking digestive-aid tablets, which contain ingredients such as betaine hydrochloride, pepsin, and herbs. Two tablets before each meal is the usual suggested amount.

A frequently-overlooked aid to digestion is exercise. A half-hour walk in the morning before breakfast gets the blood moving, the lungs pumping, and the juices stirring. Digestion and assimilation can be much improved if we make exercise a daily habit.

Exercise also sends the blood and lymph to every cell in the body, improving the circulation and thereby improving the nutrient availability. Poor circulation can cause some tissues—particularly those of the brain, hands, and feet—to be deprived of nutrients just as though our digestion or diet were impaired or deficient. The effect is the same. Exercise increases oxygen intake and oxygen, of course, is a vital food element. Oxygen can be carried only by iron-rich blood. Since 20 percent of our oxygen supply is used by the brain, it is critical to keep up our red blood count and hemoglobin by eating plenty of iron-rich foods. Without sufficient oxygen, the brain works at a lower capacity, and all organs and body systems slow down.

WHAT YOU DON'T EAT OR DRINK
CAN SAVE YOUR LOVE LIFE

A wonderful sex life may very well depend on what you leave out of your food regimen as well as what you include.

Remember that many drugs (tranquilizers, blood pressure medications) immediately impair sexual function; others (marijuana, cocaine, heroin) cause loss of sexual interest and impotence over the longer term; still others (nicotine, caffeine, alcohol) may reduce or impair sexual function in varying degrees. Alcoholics, for example, almost always become impotent at some point because alcohol destroys testosterone, the male sex hormone. Studies have shown that nicotine impairs circulation to the pelvic area and contributes to impotence. Nicotine may also interfere with the orgasm in women.

Sugar causes a quick increase in energy, followed by a lowering of energy below the previous level. At this point, mild depression is experienced by many persons, indicating a lowering of the brain chemicals called "endorphins," which promote a sense of well-being and pleasure. For these reasons, sugar interferes with the sex life and reduces its pleasure.

Fatty, fried foods are difficult to digest and may contribute to the clogging of arteries, thus reducing blood flow and oxygen availability to the brain. This will not only lower sex interest but also the level of function and response of sensory nerves. That is, sex becomes less enjoyable.

If you want to save your love life and make it more enjoyable, you need to evaluate the food and drink that have become part of your lifestyle. Use as few drugs as possible. Ask your doctor if any of the prescription drugs you have to take will affect your sex life. Cut out or cut down on the use of alcohol, cigarettes, and coffee. As much as possible, avoid sugary foods and drinks and fried, fatty foods. Cut back on milk and wheat products. Substitute herbal teas for coffee and regular teas, juices for commercial soft drinks. If you must use sweetener, use a little honey.

GOOD HEALTH IS NOT A GIFT

Only a baby has the right to say that good health is a gift. As adults, we must realize that good health is earned. It is something we have to work for. It's an end point, a consequence, the visible and present result of right living in the past. We can have a wonderful love life and wonderful sexual activity, but the two must be built on a foundation of right living. We need to learn our historical lessons and resolve to eat foods as whole, pure, and natural as we can find them. Sometimes the flame of love just dies, because we aren't eating right. The sex drive won't run without the right fuel.

DR. JENSEN'S FOOD LAWS

There are scientific laws, moral laws, and human laws to help us live better lives and better informed lives, but no laws touch our lives more intimately or vitally than our natural food laws. Following are my Food Laws. By adhering to them every day, you can move toward a more healthy, fulfilling life.

Dr. Jensen's Food Laws

Law 1: **Our foods should be whole, pure, and natural.** Whole, with no nutrients peeled, pared, or boiled away. Pure, with no preservatives, spray residues, or chemical additives of any kind. Natural—as close to the way nature made it as possible.

Law 2: **Foods in our daily meals should be in the proper proportions.** Every day we should have 6 vegetables, 2 fruits, 1 starch, and 1 protein.

Law 3: **Our food should be 80 percent alkaline and 20 percent acid.** Most people have problems with excess acidity in their bodies. The acid-alkaline balance is very important for good health and healthy sexuality.

Law 4: **Food must be taken in sufficient variety to meet the needs of every organ, gland, and tissue in the body.**

Law 5: **Our food should be 60 percent raw.** We can get live enzymes only from raw fruits, vegetables, nuts, and seeds, which provide vitamins and minerals in the form that nature intended for us to assimilate. Raw fruits and vegetables are also high in fiber, which is necessary for proper elimination and bowel health.

Law 6: **Nature cures, but she must have the opportunity.** If you don't get enough sleep, you can't stay well, and if you don't eat right, you won't stay well. Nature does the best she can with what we give her, and there lies the secret of health— we need to give her the right things. We need to live right.

Law 7: **Avoid an excess of a few foods and avoid excess eating of all foods.** You know overeating leads to obesity which is unhealthy, but, did you know eating only a few foods regularly is just as unhealthy? Imbalanced diets create chemical imbalance and deficiency in the body, which invite disease.

Law 8: **Avoid nutrient-deficient foods and nutrient-deficient diets.** I've heard of a watermelon diet, a grape diet, a high-protein diet, and many other diets, and they are all imbalanced, all deficient in important nutrients. So are refined foods, overcooked foods, and foods grown on deficient soils. Avoid them, for health's sake.

Chapter Seventeen
What Kind of Mineral Are You?

My greatest teacher, Dr. V. G. Rocine, believed that when the chemical elements are in the proper proportions in our foods, good health will follow naturally. Unfortunately, most people eat protein and carbohydrates in excess and do not eat enough of the fresh fruits and vegetables they need to provide the variety of chemical elements required. We may be made of the "dust of the earth," as Dr. Rocine liked to say, but to maintain and repair body tissues, we must get our chemicals from the vegetable and animal kingdoms, not the mineral kingdom. Rocine believed that man is at the highest level of evolution of any form of life on this planet and needs the higher evolved foods. Plants, on a lower evolutionary scale than man, can assimilate chemicals from the mineral kingdom and transform them into "living substance" that man can use for food. At the same time, Rocine believed that different types of tissue in the human body are at different levels of evolution, and these levels require different food sources.

THE BASIC CHEMICAL ELEMENTS OF MAN

The human body is 75 percent water, made of hydrogen and oxygen, but this water is always busy carrying other chemicals and nutrients, performing tasks essential to life. Human blood, which we think of as a liquid, is 78 percent water. Bone, which we think of as the most solid part of the body, is 50 percent water. The human brain, which we also think of as a solid, is 80 percent water—more liquid than the blood.

Every structure in the human body depends on nutrients carried in and wastes carried out by the blood and lymph systems, both of which are water-based liquids. The human body—from

135

the time it was a cell with a fluid interior, to an embryo in its amniotic liquid, then a human with a liquid interior again—is dependent for its life on water. Even the skin that contains it is mostly water. Hydrogen and oxygen are essential to our survival.

Of course, the human body, as well as the food we eat, is made of three basic substances—protein, carbohydrates, and fats, all of which have complex molecules (different in each case) containing hydrogen, carbon, and oxygen. Protein also contains nitrogen, and some protein contains phosphorus and sulfur.

Chemical bonding between carbon, hydrogen, and oxygen causes these three elements to act as a unit, a single molecular entity, as contrasted with free oxygen derived from the air in the lungs, or free hydrogen that joins with chlorine to form stomach acid, or pure carbon as in charcoal.

Keep in mind that every chemical element in the body performs a biological task or is part of a structure that permits tasks to be done that, when summed up over all the millions of micro-tasks done in the body each day, create health or disease. Every element has its place, every element meets a need. When our diets are deficient in some respect, certain structures become defective, or certain tasks are not done. This causes an abnormal condition to develop.

For example, a great deal of sodium, potassium, and calcium are used to neutralize the many acids that develop in the body as a consequence of normal metabolism. If these three elements were no longer made available, the acidity of the body would soon rise to a fatal level.

MINERALS MAKE THE DIFFERENCE

We don't get our minerals directly from the soil. Our bodies are not equipped to digest raw, inorganic mineral elements, so we must get them from the higher evolved sources—plants and other foods. Plants take up minerals from the soil and form organic molecular structures with them that we can digest. Similarly, animals eat plants and bring their chemical elements into new combinations and concentrations that can be utilized in human nutrition. The step from soil to plant life is a step in the evolution of minerals, and the step from plant to animal composition is another evolutionary jump.

Only the meat of young animals should be used for food. Older animals have accumulated too much toxic material in their tissues. I have advised my patients to use fresh, raw goat milk rather than cow milk, because it is more digestible and carries more nutrients. The form in which we take our minerals is very important because it determines how much of it we can digest and assimilate. We should use food sources as much as possible, and if we take mineral supplements they should be derived from natural sources.

The story of the chemical elements and their role in the human body is very important, but we are only going to summarize the main points here. My book *The Chemistry of Man* is intended for the serious students of the chemical elements who want to pursue this study in more depth.

Now let's look at the major minerals in detail. A Mineral Troubleshooting Chart closes this chapter.

Calcium—The Knitter

Calcium, "the knitter," is the most abundant element in the body. It is utilized in healing and rebuilding damaged tissue and is also required in the functioning of every cell in the body. We usually think of calcium as primarily needed to make strong bones and teeth, but it is important in sexual functioning in several ways.

Calcium aids in maintaining the right acid/alkaline balance in the blood. The acid/alkaline balance affects the production of hormones by endocrine glands, the menstrual cycle, and the fertility of both men and women. Calcium is essential to lactation and to the healthy functioning of the heart, muscles, and nerves. Stamina, energy, power, forcefulness, determination, and relaxation all require calcium in the diet and in the body.

Other effects of calcium on the sex life include steadiness of affection, prevention of overexcitement, and strength in performance. Calcium tends to keep passion under control. Glandular imbalance due to calcium deficiency can reduce both sexual interest and ability.

Women need 1,000 mg. of calcium daily to prevent osteoporosis, a calcium-depletion disease characterized by bone porosity, usually after menopause. Prior to menopause, calcium is needed by women to prevent or reduce menstrual cramps.

One of my recent discoveries is that calcium deficiency and imbalance are one component of an almost unbelievable imbalance in the average American diet. As I have pointed out, government studies have shown that the average daily diet in the United States is made up of 25 percent milk products, 29 percent wheat products, and 9 percent sugar, totaling 63 percent of the diet. The total for all three should be no more than 6 percent in a food regimen of adequate variety.

Milk these days is pasteurized and homogenized, altered from its natural form so that the calcium it contains is not as easily assimilated as calcium from fresh, whole, raw milk. Homogenized milk has been linked with atherosclerosis in several health studies.

Wheat is usually milled, resulting in significant nutrient losses, but that is not its most serious problem. The gluten in wheat products may cause celiac disease, defined in Taber's *Cyclopedic Medical Dictionary* as, "Intestinal malabsorption characterized by diarrhea, malnutrition, bleeding tendency and hypocalcemia." Hypocalcemia is calcium deficiency. The treatment for celiac disease is a wheat-free, gluten-free diet.

Sugar causes acidity in the body, which is neutralized by sodium, potassium, and calcium, a process that leaches calcium from the body. With sodium and calcium short, calcium tends to deposit in irritated joints as spurs and bumps.

Therefore, we can conclude that all three foods—wheat, milk, and sugar—contribute to calcium shortages and problems for Americans. On the other hand, the oldest, healthiest people in the world, including those in the Russian Caucasus, the Hunza Valley, and Turkey, have calcium-rich diets. I personally visited and spoke to many of these people, and most of them were still sexually active at well over 100 years old.

For proper assimilation and use in the body, calcium should be taken together with magnesium, phosphorus, and vitamins A, D, and C. It is difficult to get the right combinations and ratios in supplement form, so try to meet your basic calcium needs from food sources. Because most Americans use far too much milk in the diet, I recommend limiting consumption to a little raw milk (preferably fresh raw goat milk), yogurt, and cheese, even though milk products are high in calcium. Other high calcium foods are raw nuts and seeds (ground fine, made into seed and nut butters or into seed-or-nut-milk drinks), whole grains, green vegetables (especially kale), lentils, rice polishings, onions, parsnips, eggs, meat, and fish.

Persons who are calcium-dominant in their body chemistry are big-boned, strong physically, and strong-willed. Their hands are often large. These people tend to overwork and appear overly serious. They are slow to anger, slow in movement, slow to laugh. They are sexually dynamic. Slightly more women than men are calcium types.

Silicon—The Magnetic Element

Silicon is called the magnetic element because when it is in adequate supply in a person, that person is magnetic and attractive to others. An enjoyable sex life is impossible without silicon. The outer sheaths of the nerves throughout the body and brain need silicon. The hair, skin, and nails are dull and lifeless without silicon. This element makes us want to move, to get up and get going, to live in joy and happiness. Silicon will give you "the skin you love to touch." The best sources of silicon are oat straw tea, sprouts, rice polishings, and whole grains.

Silicon-types are quick, graceful, and animated in movement, tall and slender in build. Their faces are pleasant, open, optimistic, and they are fun-loving. Silicon people love to dance, are full of life and energy. Overspending is common. The silicon person is the most popular chemical type, with a great deal of sex appeal. This type must be careful not to live too fast or loose, because silicon people burn out suddenly and seldom recover their old spark of life.

Sodium—The Youth Element

Sodium is known as the youth element because it is necessary to keep our joints and ligaments flexible, and many people say, "You are only as young as your joints." Sodium is an acid neutralizer, used extensively in the digestive organs, blood, and lymph. Together with potassium, sodium is involved in nerve conduction. (Sodium, potassium, calcium, and magnesium all assist in neutralizing acids in the body, in maintaining the integrity of cell membranes and the electromagnetic potential of tissues.)

All body fluids carry sodium salts, including sexual fluids. While sodium is not specifically involved in human sexuality, it is so widely needed and used in the body that sex would be impossible without it. Table salt, which is sodium chloride, is not a good source of sodium because it isn't a food source. The best sources of sodium include veal joint broth, goat milk, okra, and celery.

Sodium people are restless, ready for action, often on the go. Their bodies are slender, of medium height, animated and expressive, capable of great strength and endurance but subject to sudden breakdown under high or long-term stress. Their nerve force is strong, their passions are intense, and they tend to be idealistic. The sodium type is often attractive and very appealing to the opposite sex and popular with the same sex.

Potassium—The Great Alkalizer

Potassium, like sodium, doesn't have any specifically striking functions, but it is used everywhere in the body, particularly in the heart and muscle tissue to regulate the electric potential shifts that make our muscles respond properly to the brain's directives. Without enough potassium, the heart and muscles do not work correctly, and nerve messages are impaired.

Potassium affects human sexuality by insuring healthy nerve and muscle activity, and by helping maintain the right acid/alkaline balance for hormone production in the endocrine glands. Without sufficient potassium in your diet, you would be too weak and uncoordinated to perform sexually even if the desire were present. Vitality, strength, coordination, rhythmic movement—all are aided by potassium.

The best potassium foods are blackstrap molasses, soybeans, dried fruits, bananas, raw nuts and seeds, lima beans, rice bran, wheat bran, wheat germ, parsley, lentils, spinach, avocados, and lean meat. (Cutting down on salt, sugar, coffee, and alcohol will help conserve potassium in the body.)

The potassium type of person is diplomatic, with a wonderful sense of humor; positive in attitude; aggressive; and hard working. Potassium people love to eat, drink, and be merry, and it is relatively common for them to go to excess. Unless they exercise restraint toward food, drink, and moral temptation, they may easily overdo and lose their attractive gusto for life and their popularity with others. A potassium person makes an enjoyable sex partner.

Iron—The Frisky Horse Element

Iron and oxygen together are Nature's two frisky horses in the body. Iron is part of all red blood cells, and picks up oxygen in the lungs to be used elsewhere in the body. Iron, in other words, is essential to life, as is oxygen. In addition to its importance in the blood, iron is present in enzymes that take part in cell respiration. Some iron is stored in the muscle tissue.

Anemia, often due to iron deficiency, is nearly always accompanied by fatigue and loss of interest in sex. In a sense, adequate iron is vital to an enjoyable sex life, even though it is only indirectly related to the sexual system and its functions. Iron-rich blood is basic to the process of energy production, vitality, and "feeling sexy." Among my patients who have reported active, satisfying love lives, I have always found a high red blood cell count and high hemoglobin. I know that iron is very important to a good love life.

Only a fraction of the iron in foods is absorbed. There must be trace amounts of copper, manganese, and cobalt in foods for iron to be utilized by the body. Iron absorption is increased in the presence of vitamin C and chlorophyll from green vegetables. The best sources of iron include liver and other organ meats, egg yolk, green leafy vegetables, almonds, asparagus, fish, poultry, black raspberries, bing cherries, prunes, raisins, and apricots.

There is no iron-dominant personality type.

Oxygen—The Life Giver

By weight, **oxygen** makes up 75 percent of the average human body. In comparison, it is found to be 80 percent of plants, 50 percent of minerals, 20 percent (by volume) of the air, and 89 percent of the water on planet earth. It is the only chemical element that enters the body in a "free state" from the air as well as in various chemical combinations in the foods and liquids we drink. It is the most important element in life.

Because oxygen is essential to respiration, it is essential to all life processes that contribute to human sexuality. The brain uses 20 percent of all oxygen that enters the body, indicating the importance of oxygen to brain center functioning. As sexual excitement increases, the breathing rate increases, possibly due to increased need for oxygen by brain centers that are directly and indirectly involved.

Air is a sufficient source of oxygen to meet all body needs. A relatively small amount is taken in foods and liquids.

Sulfur—The Heating Element

Sulfur is the element that supplies the spark to life, the twinkle in the eye, the quickness to the step. Sulfur people, we could say, "Are more fun!" Without enough sulfur foods in the diet, sex could become a dull, boring, routine affair! Passion would not exist without sulfur, and it affects men and women at their deepest levels.

Along with phosphorus, silicon, and manganese, sulfur is a brain and nerve element. Sulfur helps keep the skin young and flexible, promotes healthy liver function, affects hair color, and keeps us looking and acting younger. Sulfur is a cleanser and helps keep the sexual system and the rest of the body free of impurities. It helps "drive" the proper nutrients to the brain.

The best sources of sulfur: egg yolks, onions, garlic, leeks, cauliflower, broccoli, and Brussels sprouts. Others are asparagus, cabbage, kale, figs, parsnips, radishes, spinach, and turnips.

The sulfur-dominant person is usually physically attractive, well-proportioned, vivacious and lively, an extrovert among friends, an introvert among strangers. The mind is active, and this person is sensitive, with superior judgment concerning the arts, beauty, and religion. This person is more influenced by emotion and intuition than reason. The sulfur type can be fickle in life—filled with stormy passion and desire one minute, entirely indifferent the next.

Phosphorus—The Light Bearer

Phosphorus is essential to brain and nerve activity, which is, in turn, essential to human sexuality. No phosphorus; no sex life. It's that simple. Fortunately, phosphorus is seldom in short supply in most diets, although its most valuable food form is deficient in most diets. Lecithin is the most valuable form of phosphorus, and it is lost when foods are cooked at over the boiling temperature of water—212°F.

Let's start by clearing up some terms in the health literature that could be confusing. Vitellin contains phosphorus. So does lecithin. So does acetylcholine. Now, vitellin is the part of the egg yolk that contains the lecithin, and acetylcholine is possibly the most important ingredient of lecithin. Acetylcholine is a neurotransmitter necessary for proper brain function, and choline is also essential for sexual arousal.

As much as 80 percent of the male sex fluid is lecithin, but lecithin is also essential as part of nerve coating in the brain that helps keep out toxins and enhance nerve transmission.

Phosphorus is nicknamed "The Light Bearer" because of the speed of nerve conduction, which we can compare figuratively to the speed of light. Phosphorus is responsible, according to Rocine, for intelligence in man. The highest evolved phosphorus, found in eggs and meat, is needed by the brain. Bone phosphorus can come from vegetable sources.

The best sources of phosphorus and lecithin for the brain, glands, and nerves are egg yolks, codfish roe, seafood, and raw milk products. Meat, fish, and poultry, if not overcooked, may retain some phosphorus or even lecithin, but we must keep in mind that cooking over 212°F (boiling temperature) destroys lecithin. Eggs must be boiled or poached, not fried.

For building the bones, muscles, and other body tissues, phosphorus from seeds, nuts, whole grains, rice polishings, wheat bran, legumes, cabbage, corn, and other vegetable sources is perfectly adequate.

The phosphorus-dominant person is predominantly mental, intellectual, often creative, perhaps with gifts in the arts—drama, creative writing, painting, or music. This type would rather read a book or play a game of chess than go for a walk or learn to ski. Phosphorus-dominant people are often fascinating companions but must be encouraged to eat properly and exercise, or they grow flabby and lack sparkle.

Iodine—The Metabolizer

Iodine is another of those chemical elements—like iron and oxygen—that we couldn't do without. Iodine is used chiefly by the thyroid gland, which controls the metabolism of the body. Iodine helps regulate the body's production and expenditure of energy; and affects the efficiency of thought, the functioning of the speech center in the brain, and even the growth of hair, nails, skin, and teeth. Iodine does all these things (and more), because it is an essential chemical element in a hormone called thyroxine produced by the thyroid.

Iodine deficiency may cause nervousness, irritability, depression, lack of energy, and calcium-related problems, since iodine helps control blood levels of calcium. We find that the thyroid is called "the emotional gland," because it is so sensitive to emotional stress, which can rapidly deplete available stores of iodine. According to Dr. Broda Barnes in his book, *Hypothyroidism, The Unsuspected Illness*, 40 percent of Americans show evidence of underactive thyroids. An underactive thyroid can result in sterility, loss of sex drive, menstrual problems, depression, and other problems interfering with a satisfactory sex life. To normalize thyroid function, it is as important to normalize the emotional life as it is to get enough iodine-rich foods. I have known cases in which infertility was corrected by adding iodine foods to the diet.

Iodine is best taken in food form rather than in iodized salt. I recommend seafood, dulse, kelp, pineapple, and foods grown near the ocean. If you have to have salt on your food, use a little sea salt (but notice that most sea salt lacks iodine). Iodine aids in the control of calcium, silicon, and magnesium in the body.

There is no iodine chemical type.

Magnesium—The Relaxer

Magnesium not only aids in muscle relaxation, it is important in protein synthesis and generating energy from foods. Magnesium foods, such as yellow fruits and vegetables, are nature's laxatives and are wonderful for bowel health.

To enjoy life and lovemaking, we must be relaxed enough to make the most of each occasion and to keep a sense of humor and proper perspective. When a stressful lifestyle keeps a person wound up tight as a spring, joy seems to depart both from life and sex. In the sex life, too much tension spoils the enjoyment, while a relaxed and expectant attitude increases it. Magnesium, in my view, enhances our ability to focus on pleasing our partner instead of being anxious about our own performance.

Magnesium is found in high chlorophyll-rich foods such as leafy green vegetables, yellow cornmeal, raw nuts and seeds, wheat germ, whole grains, seafood, kelp, dulse, legumes, milk, and meat.

There is no magnesium personality type.

Manganese—The Love Element

In cases of **manganese** deficiency, mother rats refused to feed or care for their young and even attacked them on occasion. When manganese was available in the diet, the mother rats took excellent and even tender care of their young. So, manganese is called the mother love element. Needed in many enzyme reactions and by the brain and nerves, manganese is essential in human sexuality. The proper upkeep of all brain centers, not just the sex center, is necessary to healthy sexuality.

Manganese deficiency may cause mental problems or nerve disorders, forgetfulness, confusion, and ringing in the ears, for example. The temper may be short, poor judgment may be evident, and paranoia may appear. There is not likely to be much interest in the sex life when manganese is lacking.

In general, manganese is found in the same foods that are rich in iron—whole grains, green vegetables, egg yolks, raw nuts and seeds (Missouri black walnuts, especially), pineapple, apples, and apricots.

No manganese personality type is known.

Trace Elements (Micronutrients)

Chromium helps regulate blood sugar levels, which determine available energy. Chromium deficiency, according to experts, is relatively common in the United States because of its shortage in the soil. Best sources: Seafood, meats, whole grains, corn oil.

Cobalt is an essential chemical element in vitamin B-12, needed to make red blood cells, take care of the nerves, and activate a number of important enzymes. Best sources: Seafood, meat, milk products, Sun chlorella, seaweed.

Copper helps form red blood cells and hemoglobin by boosting iron assimilation. Best sources: Organ meats, green vegetables, raw nuts and seeds, whole grains.

Germanium is relatively new to nutritional researchers, although its health benefits were discovered about three decades ago by the late Dr. Kazuhiko Asai of Tokyo, whom I knew for many years. Organic germanium (germanium sesquioxide) alleviates mood disorders associated with loss of sex drive, enhances the disease-prevention power of the immune system, and improves bowel function. Germanium is said to have an effect in reducing cholesterol and helping to fight allergies; it has been used to treat degenerative disease.

The key to germanium's effectiveness is said to be its ability to oxygenate tissue, which stimulates the reversal of many degenerative tissue changes. Best sources: Garlic, ginseng, aloe vera, comfrey, and leafy, green vegetables.

Selenium works with vitamin E to promote fertility and to delay oxidation of unsaturated fatty acids. It also helps keep skin soft, elastic, young looking. Best sources: Bran or germ of cereal grains, broccoli, onions, tomatoes, ocean fish.

Zinc is needed by the prostate gland and spermatozoa as well as dozens of other organs, processes, and substances made in the body. It appears to play an important role in the proper maintenance of the female- as well as male sexual system. Studies have shown that deficiency can cause sterility. Zinc deficiency may be related to loss of sex drive. I believe that zinc is one of the most important chemical elements in our sex lives, affecting both men and women.

Because soils all over the world are low in zinc content, supplementation of 25 mg. per day may be advisable for all adults.

Foods high in zinc include organ meats, oysters, fish roe, eggs, whole cereal grains, and raw nuts and seeds (especially raw pumpkin seeds). Calcium supplements drive zinc levels down and extra zinc should be taken.

There is no zinc-dominant type.

Mineral Troubleshooting Chart

Mineral	Source	Function
Calcium	Whole raw milk, yogurt, cheese, raw nuts and seeds, whole grains, green vegetables (especially kale).	Maintains acid/alkaline balance; aids function of heart, muscles, and nerves; helps form bone.
Silicon	Oat straw tea, sprouts, rice polishings, whole grains.	Protects and strengthens nerves, hair, skin, nails.
Sodium	Veal joint broth, goat milk, okra, celery.	Aids function of digestive and lymphatic systems; component of blood; maintains nerve conduction and electromagnetic potential of tissues.
Potassium	Blackstrap molasses, soybeans, dried fruits, bananas, raw seeds and nuts, lima beans, rice and wheat bran, wheat germ, parsley, lentils, spinach, avocados, meat.	Electrochemical balance of tissues of heart and muscle.
Iron	Organ meats, egg yolk, green leafy vegetables, almonds, fish, asparagus, poultry, bing cherries, black raspberries, prunes, raisins, apricots.	Component of red blood cells; transports oxygen to lungs; aids in cell respiration.
Phosphorus	Brain: Egg yolks, codfish roe, seafood, raw milk. Bones: Vegetables, seeds and nuts, whole grains, rice polishings, wheat bran, legumes, cabbage, corn.	Essential to brain and nerve function.
Oxygen	Air, small amounts of solid and liquid food.	Not a mineral. Most important element of life.

Mineral Troubleshooting Chart (continued)

Mineral	Source	Function
Sulfur	Egg yolk, onion, garlic, leeks, cauliflower, broccoli, Brussels sprouts, asparagus, cabbage, kale, figs, parsnips, radishes, spinach, turnips.	Aids function of brain and nerves; a body cleanser.
Iodine	Seafood, dulse, kelp, pineapple, foods grown near the ocean.	Fuels thyroid gland, which controls the body's metabolism.
Magnesium	Leafy green vegetables, yellow cornmeal, raw nuts and seeds, wheat germ, whole grains, seafood, kelp, dulse, legumes, milk, meat.	Aids in muscle relaxation, protein synthesis, energy production; natural laxative.
Manganese	Whole grains, green vegetables, egg yolk, raw nuts and seeds, Missouri black walnuts, pineapple, apples, apricots.	Necessary in enzyme, brain function.
Chromium (Micronutrient)	Seafood, meat, whole grains, corn oil.	Aids in regulation of blood sugar levels.
Cobalt (Micronutrient)	Seafood, meat, milk products, Sun chlorella, seaweed.	Aids in formation of red blood cells, function of enzymes and nerves.
Copper (Micronutrient)	Organ meats, green vegetables, raw nuts and seeds, whole grains.	Aids in formation of red blood cells and hemoglobin.
Germanium (Micronutrient)	Garlic, ginseng, aloe vera, comfrey, green leafy vegetables.	Aids in function of immune system and bowels; may help alleviate mood disorders.

Mineral Troubleshooting Chart (continued)

Mineral	Source	Function
Selenium (Micronutrient)	Cereal brans and germs, broccoli, onions, ocean fish, tomatoes.	Works with vitamin E to delay oxidation of fatty acids and promote fertility.
Zinc	Organ meats, oysters, fish roe, whole grain cereals, raw nuts and seeds (especially pumpkin seeds).	Maintains health level of sexual system in both males and females.

Chapter Eighteen
Vitamins for a Zestful Sex Life

A lot of people say they'd like to have a super sex life, but it all boils down to the question, "Are you willing to work for it?" In a world where most people would choose a twinkie over an apple, you'll have to be the one who has the wisdom and willpower to choose the apple. In a world increasingly addicted to TV, you and your mate will have to come up with the willpower to go out on a nature walk or bicycle ride. Why? Because you can't have a super sex life unless you treat your body with the kind of love and respect that we're discussing.

We're not talking about a six-week diet in this book; we're considering a life-long program of better nutrition. We will not be advocating a three-month exercise program here to take off two inches from the waist; we're pushing for regular exercise every day of our lives! A foundation of correct nutrition and regular exercise as I am describing it is necessary before we can begin to think about a super sex life.

Most of us do not realize how foods affect our moods, feelings, energy level, and behavior. When we get down in the dumps, we don't automatically say, "Gosh, I must not have been eating right." On the other hand, when we're feeling on top of the world we don't stop to think, "I'd like to feel this good more often."

We don't relate how we feel to what we've been eating, but foods, vitamins, and minerals can make all the difference in the world between a so-so love life and the kind of love life that makes you smile every time you think about it.

We have seen how minerals affect us sexually and how a particular mineral dominance in a person's body chemistry can give rise to a particular type of physique and personality. We have seen also that specific tissues, glands, and organs require certain minerals to function properly. Over the years it has become increasingly evident to me that many people who think they have sex problems are actually victims of poor nutrition. They don't have sex problems. They have food problems. And food problems can be solved.

Just as specific minerals are needed for sexual vitality, so are specific vitamins. In almost every case our vitamins should come from eating well-balanced meals, not from vitamin supplements. (There are a few exceptions as I mention later.) The point is, even though scientists do not fully understand how some of the more complex vitamins work in the body, we do know that they are necessary to living healthy, sexually-fulfilling lives. And we also know that all we need do (unless we have special inherent weaknesses), is to select a variety of foods from the different food groups. I suggest you simply follow my Master Feeding Program (as detailed in Chapter Twenty-Two).

Now let's look at the vitamin groups in detail. A Vitamin Troubleshooting Chart closes this chapter.

Vitamin A (Retinol)

Vitamin A cannot be synthesized by the body and is necessary for normal reproduction. A deficiency of this vitamin results in atrophy of the testicles and ovaries of male and female rats, resulting in sterility in both. In male rats, sperm formation declines. In pregnant female rats, the fetus may be reabsorbed. Lack of vitamin A is believed to result in impaired production of sex hormones. The health of mucous membranes such as the nasal, respiratory, and vaginal membranes depend on vitamin A. When deficient in this vitamin, such tissues become vulnerable to inflammation and infection. Vitamin A is also needed for soft, beautiful skin. Deficiency may be indicated by dry, scaly skin.

The main food sources of vitamin A are fish, fish liver oils, liver, animal fat, eggs, cheese, and yogurt. Pro-vitamin A, or carotene, which is converted into vitamin A in the body, is high in chorella. The best sources of pro-vitamin A are green leafy vegetables, broccoli, peas, yams, sweet potatoes, carrots, and yellow fruit such as cantaloupe, peaches, and apricots. Herbs rich in vitamin A include but are not limited to parsley, mint, alfalfa, and dandelion.

Studies have shown that when vitamin A and vitamin E are taken together, the effect of each is greater. Overcooking destroys vitamin A. Main storage sites in the body for vitamin A are the liver, kidneys, lungs, and fatty tissue.

Vitamin B Family

All vitamins of the B-complex family are water soluble. This is why foods can be depleted of B vitamins by overcooking or by discarding the water in which they are cooked.

Vitamin B-1 is also called Thiamine. Deficiency leads to beri-beri, which affects the gastrointestinal, nervous, and cardiovascular systems. Since B-1 is essential to energy production and the metabolism of proteins, carbohydrates, and fats, deficiency of this vitamin can drain your energy and put an end to your sex life.

Caffeine destroys B-1 in the body, so heavy tea or coffee drinkers may become deficient. Symptoms of deficiency, besides loss of interest in sex, may include fatigue, apathy, slowed reflexes and alertness, anorexia, constipation, indigestion, deficiency of digestive acid in the stomach, and heart symptoms (after prolonged deficiency) such as rapid pulse. The heart muscle is weakened by lack of vitamin B-1. Some experts believe that moderate to severe vitamin B-1 deficiency affects 20 percent of all Americans.

The best food sources of B-1 include raw nuts and seeds (sunflower seeds are the highest), asparagus, beans, pineapple, soybeans, yogurt, wheat germ, whole wheat, brown rice and other whole grains, liver, lean meat, fish roe, and dulse. Most fruits have little B-1. Herbal sources include parsley, mint, dandelion, lamb's-quarters, bladderwick, and fenugreek. B-1 is most commonly found in the skeletal muscles, heart, kidneys, liver, and brain.

Vitamin B-2 is called riboflavin, first discovered in milk whey. It breaks down if exposed to ultraviolet light or alkaline solutions. B-2 deficiency is common, both due to dietary deficiency and due to factors that create an above normal need, such as arthritis, congestive heart disease, hyperthyroidism, and cancer. Stress can create temporary deficiency.

Riboflavin deficiency affects the sex life by robbing us of energy, since this vitamin is involved in the body's energy-producing cycles. Other signs of deficiency include cracks at the corners of the mouth, glossitis of the tongue, burning of the eyes, tears, fear of light, and the slow healing of wounds.

The best food sources of B-2 are milk, beef liver, kidney, heart, baby green vegetables, raw nuts and seeds, wheat germ, rice polishings, broccoli, asparagus, and soybeans. Herbal sources are alfalfa and parsley.

Vitamin B-3, called the "memory vitamin," also goes by the name of niacin. It is well-known for the flush a pure niacin supplement brings to the neck, face, ears, and other parts of the anatomy depending on how much is taken. Chronic niacin deficiency, called pellagra, produces skin eruptions, progressively severe mental problems, anorexia, and bowel problems. Pellagra is most common in parts of the world where corn is a big part of the diet.

The sex life is primarily affected by niacin deficiency through problems of the nerve and digestive systems. On the other hand, the sex life is enhanced by niacin's effect in dilating blood vessels and stimulating circulation to the extremities, including the brain.

The best food sources of B-3 are lean meat, chicken, fish, asparagus, dates, raw almonds, bran, wheat germ, rice polishings, broccoli, yogurt, and raw seeds. Herbal sources include alfalfa, parsley, and the seeds of burdock, fenugreek, dandelions, lamb's quarters, and sage.

Vitamin B-6 is also called Pyridoxine, the "nerve vitamin." It is important in the metabolism of amino acids and in brain function. B-6 is involved in making at least three neurotransmitters, one of which (epinephrine) is said to be involved in orgasm. It is seldom deficient, except in users of "the pill" and others who require estrogen supplements. Lack of B-6 in the pituitary, according to one researcher, can cause loss of sex drive. Other symptoms of B-6 deficiency are neuritis, weakness, irritability, insomnia, and a form of anemia.

The best food sources of B-6 are wheat germ, wheat bran, rice polishings, whole grains, liver, kidney, heart, raw nuts and seeds, eggs, honey, and molasses.

Pantothenic Acid, classified as a B-vitamin, is involved in the production of hemoglobin and acetylcholine, as well as synthesis of cholesterol. Like vitamins B-1 and B-2, pantothenic acid is needed for energy production. Pantothenic acid aids in forming steroid hormones, making the neurotransmitter acetylcholine, and building the hemoglobin that makes blood red. Choline is necessary for sexual arousal. Some experts say large amounts improve sexual performance. Like several other B-vitamins, it is seldom deficient because it is available in a variety of foods.

The best food sources are liver, kidney, heart, milk, eggs, whole grains, raw nuts and seeds, poultry, fish, molasses, broccoli, cabbage, and cauliflower. Pantothenic acid is found in nearly all plant or animal tissues.

Biotin (another vitamin in the B-family) is sometimes called a "micronutrient" because such a small amount is needed in human nutrition. Lack of biotin causes depression. Biotin deficiency can be caused by eating raw egg whites. Good sources of biotin include cereals, vegetables, milk, and liver.

PABA is short for para-aminobenzoic acid and is nearly always found with folic acid. PABA stimulates bowel bacteria to produce folic acid. It is said to be important to the health of bowels, hair, and skin. In an emergency, according to some experts, PABA can be converted to folic acid. There is no known direct effect of PABA on the sex life.

Folic Acid, like biotin and PABA, is a member of the B-vitamin family and is the vitamin most lacking in American diets. Folic acid was first extracted from foliage plants like spinach, which explains the origin of its name—folic/foliage. It is easily destroyed by cooking and depleted by stress.

Spontaneous abortion, fetal malformation, and anemia can be caused by folic acid deficiency, as can chromosome damage.

The best food sources of folic acid are liver, green leafy vegetables, broccoli, Brussels sprouts, raw nuts and seeds, asparagus, and sprouts. It is found in small amounts in many fruits and vegetables.

Choline deficiency has been linked to high cholesterol, obesity, high blood pressure, heart disease, arteriosclerosis, diabetes, and kidney trouble. Choline can be made in the body. It is one of the main ingredients in lecithin. Choline is needed to make an important brain neurotransmitter and is said to be required for sexual arousal.

The best food sources of choline are egg yolk, meat, poultry, fish, fish roe, soybeans, whole grains, and green vegetables.

Inositol, along with PABA and pantothenic acid, is considered a "youth vitamin." Along with choline, inositol helps keep our livers healthy, reduces blood cholesterol, and slows down hardening of the arteries. Caffeine in coffee and tea destroy inositol. Both choline and inositol are found in lecithin.

Since lecithin is needed by both the brain and sexual system (particularly in males where the sexual fluid is mostly made up of lecithin), choline and inositol are important to the human sex life.

The best food source of inositol is sesame-seed butter or tahini. Other sources are beef heart, whole grains, blackstrap molasses, soybeans, grapefruit, legumes, eggs, and fish roe. High heat destroys lecithin, so lecithin foods should be taken raw or cooked at low heat. Eggs should be poached or boiled, not fried.

Vitamin B-12 (Cobalamine) contains an atom of cobalt and is the most complex vitamin known. It is needed to synthesize DNA (nucleic acid) and myelin (the fatty substance that covers and protects the nerves), and it is essential in the metabolism of proteins, carbohydrates, and fats. Vitamin B-12 works with folic acid to prevent anemia. All cells in the body need vitamin B-12.

The sex drive is reduced when B-12-deficiency anemia is present, and nerve problems may also create sexual difficulties. Deficiency of B-12 can result from inadequate intake or utilization, increased excretion, and increased need. It may be necessary to treat the condition causing the deficiency while taking B-12 supplements to overcome it, reducing the amount taken as the body normalizes. The use of laxatives depletes B-12. This vitamin is not well absorbed when the body is deficient in iron, B-6, and calcium. Vegetarians are frequently deficient in vitamin B-12.

Symptoms of vitamin B-12 deficiency in the early stages may include fatigue, irritability, and mental slowness. As time goes on, menstrual disturbances, paleness, muscle-jerking, and mild to severe mental problems may appear. Even the early symptoms can practically destroy a person's sex life.

The best food sources of B-12 are lean meats (especially organ meats such as liver), fish, poultry, eggs, cheese, milk, yogurt, chlorella, and seaweed. Chlorella is the highest known vegetarian source of B-12.

Vitamin C (Ascorbic Acid)

Vitamin C, like the B-vitamins, is water soluble, easily lost in cooking, and very important in many ways. This vitamin promotes better absorption or use of vitamins A, B-complex, and E; iron; and calcium. Its potency is lost by exposure to air, heat, or light. Deficiency of vitamin C for a period of over four months produces scurvy, a disease that attacks the bones and joints. While scurvy is rare these days, lower levels of deficiency are not.

Vitamin C affects the sex life directly through its role in the absorption of iron, the formation of blood cells, and the metabolism of the adrenal gland, which stores large amounts of this vitamin. All these processes influence the sex life. Iron aids in oxygenation of the tissues for energy production. Blood carries oxygen, hormones, and nutrients to the organs, glands, and tissues. The adrenal glands make several hormones and neurotransmitters that influence our sex life, including a hormone involved in stimulating orgasm. Indirectly, vitamin C supports our sex lives by keeping the joints limber and active, strengthening the immune system, helping normalize blood cholesterol, protecting against stress, and detoxifying the body by removal of heavy metals and other harmful substances.

Normally, the adult body contains five grams of vitamin C. Our body's supply of vitamin C is reduced by smoking, stress, fever, aspirin, antibiotics, cortisone, sulfa drugs, exposure to the pesticide DDT, gasoline fumes, and drinking too much water. If the acid/alkaline balance of the blood shifts too much to the alkaline side, vitamin C is destroyed.

Signs of deficiency are bleeding gums, bruising easily, poor digestion, shortness of breath, nosebleeds, anemia, swollen or painful joints, and slow healing of wounds or broken bones.

The best food sources of vitamin C are acerola, strawberries, tomatoes, mangos, Brussels sprouts, avocados, and citrus fruits.

Vitamin D

Vitamin D is actually a group of hormone-like compounds, sterols designed to control calcium, aid in bone growth, and control the calcium-phosphorus balance. It is useless to take calcium supplements if you are not getting enough vitamin D, since the calcium will only be excreted. Vitamin D can be formed in the body when a certain type of cholesterol in the bloodstream flows through the capillaries near the surface of the skin and is exposed to the ultraviolet in sunlight. Or it can be taken as a supplement in the form of fish-liver oil.

There is no known direct effect of vitamin D on the human sexual system, but there may be an indirect effect through its role in controlling blood calcium and the ratio of calcium to phosphate. When vitamin D is lacking in the diet, calcium absorption goes down. Because the calcium/phosphorus ratio must be held constant, the kidneys also excrete more phosphorus. This means that dietary choline and lecithin, which contain phosphorus, may be broken down and excreted. Choline and lechithin are needed by the sexual system and by the brain for normal functioning.

Deficiency of vitamin D was once common in the United States and resulted in rickets, a children's disease characterized by leg-bone deformity and caused by inadequate calcium and phosphorus. In adults, osteomalacia may develop in place of rickets. Microfractures in the leg bones, and pain in the legs and back are common symptoms. Older adults, especially postmenopausal women, may get osteoporosis, a weakening of the bones due to lack of calcium, but this is mainly because of calcium deficiency rather than vitamin D deficiency.

The best food sources of vitamin D are fish, butter, eggs, and liver. Fish-liver oils are concentrated natural sources.

Vitamin E

Vitamin E compounds are called tocopherols, which means "to bring childbirth" in Greek, because this vitamin was first discovered to be necessary to the reproductive systems of animals.

Experts still disagree on what vitamin E compounds do, but all agree that they protect fatty acids from oxidation. Fatty acids are necessary in the production of sex hormones. Vitamins A and C are protected by vitamin E, and both are involved in healthy sexuality. Despite experiments on animals that show vitamin E's necessity in reproductive activity, no such evidence is available regarding humans. Vitamin E is believed to prevent or alleviate cardiovascular disease by some experts. Obviously, a healthy heart is an asset in an enjoyable sex life. The hormones of the pituitary and adrenal glands are protected from oxidation by vitamin E, which also aids in muscle cell respiration (and increases available energy). Some researchers feel that vitamin E slows the aging process.

This vitamin also reduces venous congestion, removes toxic materials from mucous membranes (such as in the vaginal tract), and reduces undesirable symptoms of menopause. Leucorrhea, endometriosis, and irregular menstruation are improved by vitamin E.

Vitamin E deficiency in adults in the United States has not been carefully studied, and even experts disagree on how much should be taken. The most active and beneficial form of vitamin E is alpha tocopherol. (Six other forms exist.)

Sources of vitamin E are abundant and include eggs, fish roe, cheese, sardines, liver, soybeans, leeks, cabbage, Brussels sprouts, and herbs like parsley, dill, and dandelion. Raw wheat germ and wheat germ oil are good sources (one teaspoon of wheat germ oil has about 10 I.V. of vitamin E). Raw nuts, seeds, and sprouts contain vitamin E. Nevertheless, it is hard to get all the vitamin E needed from natural sources, and many people take supplements to make sure they are getting enough.

Vitamins F and K

Vitamin F, or Essential Fatty Acids, can be easily neglected but shouldn't be. Consisting of linoleic, linolenic, and arachidonic acids (unsaturated fatty acids), vitamin F can't be made in the body and must be taken from foods.

In relation to the sex life, vitamin F is needed by the thyroid gland, adrenal glands, and prostate, as well as to manufacture prostaglandins, a group of chemical substances in the body that work together with hormones.

Vitamin F promotes calcium absorption, slows cholesterol buildup, regulates blood coagulation, aids in forming membranes, keeps hair lustrous, and moistens the skin.

Deficiency of vitamin F may result in diarrhea, weight loss, varicose veins, brittle hair, dandruff, skin disorders, problems with fat metabolism, and a lowered immune system response. The best food sources of vitamin F are raw nuts and seeds, whole grains, wheat germ, whole milk, and vegetable oils such as cottonseed, safflower, and soybean.

Vitamin K has no known relation to the sex life. Its function is to help form prothrombin, the blood-clotting factor. The best food sources are kidneys, cabbage, soybeans, spinach, and cauliflower.

VITAMINS AND YOUR DIET

Now that we have a basic understanding of the vitamin groups and how they affect our sex lives and our health in general, the next step is to plan our meals such that we are assured of getting enough of all the chemical elements and vitamins. Under the best of circumstances—in a world where a variety of foods is plentiful, affordable, and easily prepared—such assurance would be taken for granted. Even in our wealthy Western nations, however, we cannot take our diets for granted. A "progressive" civilization does not necessarily produce finer, more wholesome foods, or people who are willing to take time to enjoy their meals. Quite the contrary, it would seem that most "advanced" societies have depleted their soils, polluted their natural foods and water, and processed the vital minerals and vitamins away. We have learned to "mass-market" and "fast-food" ourselves into nutritional bankruptcy, assuming that we can compensate for months of inadequate eating by gulping vitamin supplements or magic potions.

There is no substitute for balanced foods, no shortcut to good health. If you truly want to improve your sex life—and your overall health—I suggest you take the time to follow my Master Feeding Program, detailed in Chapter Twenty-Two.

Vitamin Troubleshooting Chart

Vitamin	Source	Function
Vitamin A (Retinol)	Fish, fish-liver oils, liver, meat, eggs, cheese, yogurt.	Sex hormone production; protection of nasal, respiratory, and vaginal membranes.
Pro-Vitamin A (Carotene)	Leafy green vegetables, yellow fruits and vegetables, broccoli, peas.	Converted to vitamin A.
Vitamin B$_1$ (Thiamine)	Raw nuts and seeds, asparagus, beans, pineapple, soybeans, yogurt, wheat germ, whole grains, herbs, liver, meat, fish roe.	Energy production, aids overall metabolism.
Vitamin B$_2$ (Riboflavin)	Milk, organ meats, baby green vegetables, raw nuts and seeds, wheat germ, rice polishings, broccoli, asparagus, soybeans, herbs.	Energy production, healing of wounds.
Vitamin B$_3$ (Niacin)	Meat, chicken, fish, asparagus, dates, raw almonds, bran, wheat germ, rice polishings, broccoli, yogurt, raw seeds, herbs.	Aids circulatory and digestive system function.
Vitamin B$_6$ (Pyridoxine)	Wheat germ, wheat bran, rice polishings, whole grains, organ meats, raw nuts and seeds, eggs, honey, molasses.	Aids metabolism of amino acids; aids in brain function.

Vitamin Troubleshooting Chart (continued)

Vitamin	Source	Function
Pantothenic Acid (B vitamin Category)	Organ meats, milk, eggs, whole grains, raw nuts and seeds, poultry, fish, molasses, broccoli, cabbage, cauliflower.	Aids in production of red blood cells, steroid hormones, and overall energy.
Biotin (B vitamin Category)	Cereals, vegetables, milk, liver, raw egg white.	May alleviate symptoms of depression.
PABA (B vitamin Category)	See Folic Acid.	Involved in production of folic acid; aids function of bowels, hair, skin; nearly always found with folic acid.
Folic Acid (B vitamin Category)	Liver, leafy green vegetables, broccolie, Brussels sprouts, raw nuts and seeds, asparagus, sprouts.	Involved in maintenance of chromosomes; safeguards against anemia.
Choline (B vitamin Category)	Egg yolk, meat, poultry, fish, fish roe, soybeans, whole grains, green vegetables.	Aids in production of neurotransmitters; aids in function of circulatory system and kidney function.
Inositol (B vitamin Category)	Sesame seed butter, tahini, beef heart, whole grains, blackstrap molasses, soybeans, grapefruit, legumes, eggs, fish roe.	See Choline.
Vitamin B_{12}	Meat, organ meats, fish, poultry, eggs, cheese, milk, yogurt, chlorella, seaweed.	Aids in DNA synthesis; metabolizes proteins, carbohydrates, fats; prevents anemia.

Vitamin Troubleshooting Chart (continued)

Vitamin	Source	Function
Vitamin C	Acerola, strawberries, tomatoes, mangoes, avocadoes, Brussels sprouts.	Promotes absorption of other vitamins, iron, calcium; necessary for function of adrenal glands; protects body against stress.
Vitamins D	Fish, butter, eggs, liver, fish-liver oils.	Controls calcium levels.
Vitamin E	Eggs, fish roe, cheese, sardines, liver, soybeans, leeks, cabbage, Brussels sprouts, herbs, raw wheat germ; nuts, seeds, and sprouts.	Protects fatty acids from oxidizing; aids in sex hormone production; reduces venous congestion.
Vitamin F	Raw seeds and nuts, whole grains, wheat germ, whole milk, vegetable oils.	Aids in function of thyroid, adrenal, and prostate glands; manufactures prostaglandins; promotes calcium absorption; slows cholesterol buildup.
Vitamin K	Kidneys, cabbage, soybeans, spinach, cauliflower.	Aids in formation of Prothrombin, a blood-clotting factor.

Part Four
PUTTING IT ALL TOGETHER

Chapter Nineteen
Putting It All Together

I like to read newspaper- and magazine articles that tell about foods to which various sex-enhancing powers are attributed. Any foods that are new, rare, or exotic are likely to develop a rumored reputation of stimulating the love life. For example, tomatoes, when they were first discovered, were called "love apples" and were thought to have the power to stimulate sexual desire. Chocolate, discovered by the Aztecs, was believed to stimulate desire in that ancient culture. Oysters, perhaps because of their similarity in shape to male gonads, have long been thought to enhance sexual powers. They are high in zinc and essential to the prostate, which may give the story some credibility. Cooked sheep testicles, called "Rocky Mountain Oysters," are considered a delicacy by some in the sheep-raising country of the West.

There are, of course, many other such foods including mangoes, bananas, Mandrake root, caviar, apples, figs, and dates. Is there any substance to the claims that these foods enhance the sex life? It's very difficult to tell.

However, there are good, sensible reasons why we shouldn't rely on special foods to build up our sex life unless we build on the foundation of a balanced food regimen, regular exercise, sufficient rest, and a healthy lifestyle. If the body isn't as healthy as it should be, and you use a food that increases your sexual desire, you will be robbing the energy systems of your body to "turn on" a temporarily-hyperactive sex drive. We might call this the "play-now-pay-later" syndrome. It seems like such a good idea at the time, but we're usually sorry later when we feel the consequences.

On the other hand, if you've been following a healthy way of life and have built up a reservoir of surplus available energy, you

Chemical Elements of the Body

The average human body (160 lbs.) contains the following proportions of chemical elements:

Carbon-45 lbs.	Calcium-4 lbs.	Potassium-3 1/4 oz.
Hydrogen-15 lbs.	Phosphorus-2 lbs.	Sodium-3 oz.
Nitrogen-2 lbs.	Sulfur-3 3/4 oz.	Silicon-1 1/4 oz.
Oxygen-89 lbs.	Magnesium-3 1/2 oz.	Iron-2 oz.
Chlorine-1 3/4 lbs.	Fluorine-3 3/4 oz.	Manganese-1/2 oz.
	Iodine-1/4 oz.	

can use sexually stimulating foods (natural foods) without harm to your body or its systems and functions.

I want to emphasize that research on how extensively nutritional deficiencies affect the sex life has barely begun, and I feel that we have much more to find out about how our sex lives are dramatically affected by what we eat and don't eat. This will be demonstrated foremost, I believe, in the brain, nerves, and glands, the three most important components in the sexual system.

When men and women become sexually aroused, a great many physiological events take place, principally through the brain, nerves, and glands. Spinal nerves transmit brain messages to different parts of the body that result in tensed muscles, blood rushing into the pelvis, an increased heart rate, changes in blood pressure and breathing rate, glandular secretions, and increased excitement. As we have seen, none of these processes can take place without the availability of many chemical elements, enzymes, vitamins, prostaglandins, amino acids, neurotransmitters, and other food-derived chemical substances. Any process that lowers oxygen, glucose, or choline supplies to the brain can reduce a person's sensitivity to sexual stimulation, even to complete loss of interest.

A HOLISTIC APPROACH TO DIET

I live by a holistic philosophy of life and I take care of my patients with a holistic approach to the natural health art simply because it's a better way to live, with no hidden liabilities popping up later, as is the case with using drugs or alcohol to stimulate sexual pleasure. People who grow to depend on such things end up destroying their sex lives—and often everything else they hold dear.

The foundation for the best sex life you can possibly have is made up of a proper food regimen, regular exercise, enough rest, a positive attitude, and moral beliefs that draw the respect of others—even when they may disagree with you. Lack of moral strength and integrity is one of the greatest weaknesses in our modern society, yet no man or woman can be truly happy without it, because sex without self-respect is never satisfying to anyone. I'm not trying to preach to you about morals. I'm trying to help you achieve a great sex life; and the truth is, you can't have a great sex life without at the same time being able to love and respect yourself. Remember, also, that good sex, like good health, depends on the total harmony of the body, mind, and spirit.

To put the question in a different light, why should I show you how to have a wonderful sex life (through having a healthy body), if you don't have a healthy mind and spirit as well? You must live right, treat yourself right, and treat others as you want to be treated. Lack of morality kills and hurts, just like a disease. Sex can be very destructive—to oneself and others—if used without mental and moral guidance.

So if you enter into my program, which is intended to replace the old unsatisfactory lifestyle with a new one that you're going to live, you'll have a wonderful sex life—if you can walk the path that leads to it.

We do this not by advocating sex-enhancing foods by themselves but rather a balanced food regimen that builds the whole body—including the sexual system—and maintains a healthy mind and spirit, too. No organ or system functions by itself without visible means of support (from other organs or systems). Similarly, no organ or system can work independently of the mind, and the mind must discover its spiritual harmony. Strength and the capacity to enjoy life and health come out of this community relationship.

HOW CAN I GIVE MY WHOLE BEING WHAT IT NEEDS?

It's simple, once you understand some basic principles about your being's relationship with food, and what kinds of foods are needed to fulfill that relationship. Keep your attention on foods that build health. The rest aren't worth the bother, even if they are free.

Your body needs whole, pure, and natural foods. Whole foods are foods that haven't had any essential nutrient removed, so they contain more food value—brown rice instead of white rice, whole wheat flour instead of refined white flour, honey instead of white sugar. Pure foods are better for you than foods with chemical additives, because no chemical additive belongs in the human body. It may be harmless in itself, but it was not created by nature to go in your body, so leave it out. (It may not be harmless, especially when combined with the other chemicals inside your body.) Natural foods are unprocessed, as nature made them. Every step of processing by man involves removing something that's good for you or adding something that isn't. So we should stick to natural foods as much as possible.

We should have 60 percent of our foods (such as fruits, vegetables, nuts, and seeds) raw because we get the most food value that way. We need six vegetables, two fruits, one starch, and one protein each day—vegetables and fruits for minerals, vitamins, enzymes, and fiber; starchy food for energy; and protein for repair and building. Of these foods 80 percent should be alkaline and 20 percent acid. If you keep to the ratio of six vegetables, two fruit, and one starch and one protein, you'll be preserving the right acid/alkaline balance.

The environment of your body—the temperature, fluid volume, acid/alkaline balance (pH), blood and lymph (and the nutrients they carry), oxygenation and rapid removal of wastes—determine whether your life is going to feel like a joyful occasion or a punishment. The food you put in your body determines whether your body is going to serve you well or not.

GENERAL DIETARY PRINCIPLES

You must have variety in your foods because each organ, gland, and tissue has different nutrient needs. You not only have to feed your glands the right foods to make hormones in the right amounts, you also have to supply the chemical elements needed for glands to repair and rebuild themselves. This same principle follows for every specialized organ, gland, and tissue—including the sexual system. It has to be kept clean, supplied with energy, provided with building materials to repair itself and to make hormones, ova, sperm. Your sexual system will be made up of whatever you give your body, whether coffee and donuts, or a chef's salad. Meat, poultry, and fish should be broiled, baked, or

Dr. Jensen's Food Proportions

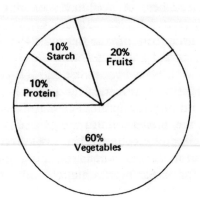

Food Proportions

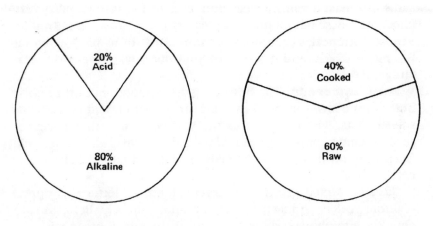

Acid/Alkaline Proportions   **Raw/Cooked Proportions**

The proportions of foods we eat each day are important to maintaining healthfulness. We should eat six vegetables, two fruits, one starch, and one protein each day. By adhering to this mix of foods, we will achieve an 80 percent alkaline/20 percent acid proportion. To further ensure we obtain optimum nutrition, 60 percent of our foods should be eaten raw.

roasted—never fried or deep-fat cooked. Cook at lower temperatures for longer times to improve flavor and reduce nutrient losses.

It's best to use low-heat, waterless cookware and cook with as little water as possible until food is barely done, not overcooked. Steaming is second best. A double boiler may be used on some occasions.

Avoid eating an excess of one or two foods and try to have at least one whole cereal grain each day. Don't fill up on meat and potatoes so you don't have room for enough vegetables. I suggest having your protein at one meal and your starch at another to increase your fruit and vegetable intake at every meal.

Meat, poultry, and fish. Buy from a reliable source and talk to the store butcher about the quality. Avoid fatty meats, including pork. Cut down on beef or cut it out altogether, and your body will thank you for it. Eat more chicken and fish. Use only white-fleshed fish with fins and scales, except for salmon which is fine despite its pink meat. Cheese is excellent.

Starches and whole grain cereals. The most nutritious form of potatoes is baked, followed by steaming (cut up with skins on). Baked yams, sweet potatoes, and squash are also very good. The best whole grains are short grain brown rice, millet, yellow cornmeal, rye, and buckwheat. Most of us have eaten far too much wheat, and it is best to limit our intake or avoid wheat altogether.

Nuts and seeds. The best nut is the almond, but other good nuts are the Missouri black walnut, the chestnut, and other hard-shelled nuts. The best seed is the sesame seed. Other excellent seeds include sunflower, pumpkin, melon, chia, and fenugreek. Keep in mind that nuts and seeds are high in fats and should be eaten raw.

Salads. Mixed green (mix several kinds of lettuce, chopped scallions, celery, spinach leaves, cut-up cucumber, slices, tomato chunks); a rainbow salad is the same as the mixed green with the addition of grated zucchini, parsnips, raw carrots, and raw beets (the grated amount should be about the size of a golf ball); cole slaw (chopped cabbage, celery seed, chopped onions); mixed fruit (with nuts, raisins, and yogurt dressing); shredded carrots and raisins; potato salad; and Waldorf salad (apples, raisins, and nuts).

Salad dressings. Blue cheese, roquefort, vinegar and oil, avocado, nut butter, mayonnaise, oil with lemon and honey.

Legumes. The best legumes are lentils, lima beans, soybeans, garbanzos, black beans, split peas, and pinto beans. (Soak overnight before cooking to reduce production of gas.)

Sprouts are best taken raw in salads or alone. Seeds and nuts should be converted to "milk drinks" or "butters" before being used, because most people don't chew them well enough to get all the good out of them. Another way is to grind them fine in a coffee grinder or blender, then sprinkle them on other foods such as salads, soups, and cooked vegetables. For nut or seed milk drinks, soak 1/4 cup of raw almonds, sunflower seeds, pumpkin seeds or hulled sesame seeds in apple or pineapple juice overnight. Add to 2 cups distilled water or apple juice in blender and run on high until well blended. Drink as is, or strain through 2 layers cheesecloth or wire strainer. (If you use unhulled sesame seeds, always run the blenderized liquid through cheesecloth or a strainer.) Nut and seed butters can be made with raw nuts and seeds in a Champion juicer.

I realize, of course, that my general dietary recommendations and basic principles for achieving good health and improving your sex life will only go so far. You need menus and directions for the kitchen, a recipe for better meals, better sex, and better health. In the next chapter, I share with you the meal programs that have been used successfully at my ranch for many years. For some of you, my meal programs may be quite a departure from the high-fat, high-cholesterol, low-fiber foods to which you have grown accustomed. To you I say, "Welcome. Eat, drink, and be healthy."

Chapter Twenty

Sample Daily Meals and My Master Formula

Here in a brief outline form is my Sample Daily Meal Program. You should fill in specific foods to your tastes, availability, and needs. You can begin my program gradually or all at once, but if your mate or children rebel, you will have to ease them into the plan more slowly. Then your loved ones can discover for themselves how much better life can be when they enjoy good foods—and good health—each day.

Sample Daily Meal Program

Breakfast

½ Starch portion

½ Protein portion

Health drink

---

10 a.m. Snack

Juice, broth, or herbal tea

Lunch

3 Vegetables (cooked, raw, or salad)

1/2 Starch portion

Health drink, Fruit dessert

3 p.m. Snack

Juice, broth, or herbal tea

Dinner

3 Vegetables (cooked, raw, or salad)

1/2 Protein portion

Health drink, Fruit dessert

INSTRUCTIONS TO THE KITCHEN STAFF

Here are the specific instructions my kitchen staff at the Ranch has followed for many years in meal planning and preparation.

Breakfast

Fruit: One fresh fruit and one dried fruit. Also, prunes every morning with juice or water.

Beverages: Milk, if desired. Whey. Tea: Three different teas should be served during the day. Five different kinds should be kept on hand in the kitchen.

Cereal: Yellow cornmeal (twice a week). Muesli (twice a week), Rye, Oatmeal, Millet. Always serve five different ones during the week.

Eggs: Soft and hard-boiled

Sunday mornings: O.K. to serve cornmeal hotcakes.

Bread and Butter: Toaster in working order.

Supplements: Wheat germ, rice polishings, flaxseed meal, sesame seed meal.

Lunch

Salad Bar: Dish of olives, Waldorf salad (peel apples) once or twice a week. Gelatin mold (shredded carrot and pineapple) once or twice a week. Stuffed celery (with almond or cashew butter) twice a week. Stuffed dates (almond or cashew butter) once a week. Carrot and cashew salad (made in a Champion juicer) once a week. Carrot and pea salad (cheese) once a week. Cole slaw once a week.

Always serve: Finely-shredded carrots, beets, turnips; carrot sticks; celery sticks; sliced tomatoes; sliced cucumbers; sliced green peppers. Anything else in season, used raw: Jicama, zucchini, summer squash, onions (small), parsley, watercress, endive. Serve alfalfa sprouts daily, and other sprouts occasionally.

Salad dressings: Avocado; cheese and yogurt; nut butter; cottage cheese with blue cheese and yogurt; oil, vinegar, and honey.

Vegetables: Two (cooked): Use one vegetable from under the ground and one vegetable from above the ground. One bland vegetable must be served, such as: beets, squash (yellow neck, banana, winter, zucchini), peas, carrots, string beans, wax beans, spinach, asparagus. Other vegetables may be of the sulphur-type (but do not have to be). These are: cabbage, cauliflower, Brussels sprouts, onions, broccoli, turnips, kohlrabi. Steamed onions may be served (creamed with parsley) once a week as a separate dish. Do not put onions in soups, loaves, etc.

Starch: Brown rice (twice a week), baked potato (twice a week), lima beans, cornbread, yams.

Beverages: Milk, whey, buttermilk, tea, nut milk drink (once a week), Doctor's drink (once a week).

Dinner

Protein: Note: A meat meal is to be served no more than three times a week. Meat (lean, no fat, no pork). Use: Chicken, turkey, beef, beef roast, meatloaf, lamb roast; fish (baked and served on Friday) including ocean white fish, halibut, bass, trout, salmon loaf. On other nights, instead of meat or fish, use nut loaf, cheese souffle, cottage cheese loaf, spinach loaf, eggplant and cheese loaf.

Vegetables: Two cooked vegetables and salad, as for Lunch.

Fruit and cheeses: Two nights a week. Assorted cheeses: Swiss, Jack, cheddar, cottage cheese, and yogurt. Assorted fresh fruits: Three kinds, such as melons, apples, persimmons, pears, cherries, berries, oranges, apricots, peaches.

Nuts and Dates: Assorted varieties.

Crackers: Ry-Krisp, Ak-mak, or sesame.

Desserts: Natural desserts allowed three times a week. However, they are not recommended.

Juices: Fresh fruit- and vegetable juices.

SAMPLE MENUS

For an idea of what an average week's meal plan would be like, following is a list of seven breakfasts, lunches, and dinners.

Menu One

Breakfast	Lunch	Dinner
Museli with bananas and dates	Vegetable salad	Diced celery and carrots
Oat straw tea	Baby lima beans	Steamed spinach, waterless cooked
Add eggs, if desired or sliced peaches with cottage cheese	Baked potato	Puffy omelet
Herb tea	Spearmint tea	vegetable broth

Menu Two

Breakfast	Lunch	Dinner
Fresh figs	Vegetable salad (with health mayonnaise)	Salad
Cornmeal cereal	Steamed asparagus	Cooked beet tops
Shavegrass tea	Very ripe bananas or steamed unpolished rice	Meat or fish
Add eggs or nut butter or raw applesauce and blackberries	Vegetable broth or herb tea	Tomato Sauce
		Cauliflower
		Comfrey tea

Menu Three

Breakfast	Lunch	Dinner
Reconstituted dried peaches	Raw salad plate w/French dressing	Cottage cheese, cheese sticks
Millet cereal	Baked zucchini and okra	Apples, peaches, grapes, nuts
Alfa-mint tea	Corn on the cob	Apple concentrate cocktail
Add eggs, cheese or nut butter or	Ry-Krisp crackers	
Sliced nectarines and apples	Buttermilk or herb tea	
Yogurt		

Menu Four

Breakfast	Lunch	Dinner
Prunes or any reconstituted dried fruit	Salad	Salad
Brown rice with cinnamon and honey or reconstituted raisins	Baked green pepper stuffed with eggplant and tomatoes	Steamed chard, baked eggplant
Oat straw tea	Baked potato and/or bran muffin	Poached fresh salmon
Grapefruit and kumquats	Carrot soup or herb tea	Persimmon whip (optional)
Poached eggs		Alfa-mint tea

Menu Five

Breakfast	Lunch	Dinner
Slices of fresh pineapple with shredded coconut	Salad	Salad
Buckwheat cereal	Steamed turnips and turnip greens	Yogurt and lemon dressing
Peppermint tea/or baked apple, persimmons	Baked yam	Steamed mixed greens, beets
Chopped raw almonds	Catnip tea	Tofu with soy sauce
Acidophilus milk		Leek soup, herb tea

Menu Six

Breakfast	Lunch	Dinner
Cornmeal Cereal	Salad w/lemon and	Salad
Reconstituted dried	olive oil dressing	Cooked string beans,
fruit	Steamed whole barley	baked summer
Dandelion coffee or	Cream of celery soup	squash
herb tea	Steamed chard	Carrot and cheese loaf
	Herb tea	Cream of lentil soup
		or lemongrass tea
		Fresh peach gelatin
		w/almond-nut cream

Menu Seven

Breakfast	Lunch	Dinner
Cooked applesauce	Carrot and cashew	Salad
with raisins	salad	Diced carrots and
Shavegrass tea or	Steamed broccoli	peas, steamed
cantaloupe and	Brown rice	Tomato aspic
strawberries	Vegetable broth	Roast leg of lamb
Cottage cheese		w/mint sauce
		Herb tea

MASTER FORMULA FOR MEN AND WOMEN

The preceding mini-dictionary of foods and herbs that support and enhance the reproductive systems may be used with my Master Feeding Program in Chapter Nineteen to help balance your body systems in accordance with the wholistic perspective we have previously described. I am also not opposed to the use of a high-quality, multi-vitamin supplement used with extra niacin to stimulate circulation.

You should be exercising daily (see Chapter Twenty-two), skin brushing, keeping your body clean inside and out, and trying your best to maintain a total harmony of your mind, body, and spirit.

To strengthen and enhance the reproductive system, brain, nerves, and endocrine glands, I have developed my Master Formula for Men and my Master Formula for Women. Each was developed specifically for use with my Master Feeding Program. You may need to take a little more or a little less of a particular supplement because individual needs vary. However, taking a mega-dose of my supplement at any one time will not help. Simply follow directions.

Master Formula For Women

Master Formula	Other Useful Supplements
Dong Quai (3 times daily)	Cod liver oil (vitamins A & D)
Sun Chlorella (5 tablets, 3 times daily)	Rice bran syrup (B vitamins)
Nova Scotia dulse (3 times daily)	Bee pollen (many vitamins, lecithin, minerals)
Lecithin (tbsp. daily)	Royal jelly (hormone-like substances, lecithin)
Sesame seed butter (tbsp. daily)	Alfalfa sprouts (silicon, vitamins)
Wheat germ oil (tsp. 3 times daily)	Kyolic tablets (deodorized garlic)
Lactobacillus acidophillus (3 times daily)	Pumpkin seeds (lecithin, zinc, vitamin E)
	Aloe vera (enzymes, vitamins)
	Echinacea, oat straw tea, fenugreek, red raspberry

Menstrual Problems: The following herbs have been recommended for menstrual problems: licorice root, black cohosh, and squaw vine. (Instead of black cohosh, black hawthorne or blessed thistle may be used.)

Infertility Problems: For correction of some infertility problems, the following have been recommended: fo-ti tieng, false unicorn, saw palmetto, vitamin E-400 I.U. each meal, niacin 100 mg. each meal. (Always see your doctor about fertility problems.)

Master Formula For Men

Master Formula	Other Useful Supplements
Ginseng (3 times daily)	Cod liver oil (vitamins A & D)
Nova Scotia dulse (3 times daily)	Rice bran syrup (B-complex)
Gotu Kola (3 times daily)	Bee pollen (vitamins, lecithin, minerals, silicon)
Sun Chlorella (5 tablets, 3 times daily)	Royal jelly (hormone-like substance, lecithin)
Lecithin (tbsp. daily)	Alfalfa sprouts (silicon, vitamins)
Pumpkin seeds (tbsp. ground fine daily)	Kyolic tablets (deodorized garlic)
Lactobacillus acidophillus (3 times daily)	Wheat germ or wheat germ oil (vitamin E)
	Aloe vera (tonic)
	Echinacea, oatstraw tea, fenugreek

Infertility Problems: The following have been recommended for some infertility problems in men: saw palmetto, sarsaparilla, niacin (100 mg. with each meal), vitamin E (400 I.U. with each meal).

Chapter Twenty-One
Special Foods for Special Problems

One of the most encouraging and fascinating facts about the human body is that chemical replacement is constantly taking place. No matter how much a particular organ, gland, or tissue has deteriorated, we can replace that underactive, toxic-laden tissue with new tissue made form the right foods with exactly the right chemical elements.

We're all familiar with the basic division of the body into specialized systems (such as the respiratory- and nervous systems), each of which is further divided into specialized organs, glands, and tissues. Each of these organs, glands, and tissues performs a unique function in the body and requires a unique set of chemical elements to be healthy and work efficiently. This knowledge helps us to identify specific nutrient needs when certain organs are ailing, so we can develop a balanced nutritional regimen that will begin to take care of the problem at its root. (See Nutrient Chart that follows.)

Researchers have not pinned down all of the chemical elements and more complex nutrients essential to the maximum-level functioning of each part of the human sexual system, but we do know enough to design a balanced food regimen to produce a peak physical fitness for optimum sexuality. Most of us don't have to worry about reaching that "maximum" level of health because we are exposed to so many contaminants and pollutants on a daily basis that our bodies cannot expel them any faster than they accumulate. Most Americans do not eat balanced, nutritious meals that are necessary for good sex and good health. Nevertheless, you can do a lot better than the average person and you will, if you use what you are learning in this book.

Key Nutrient Requirements

Nutrient	Organ or Gland
Calcium	Bones
Iodine	Thyroid
Silicon	Skin
Zinc	Prostate
Iron	Blood
Potassium	Muscles
Phosphorus	Brain
Sodium	Stomach and Bowel

For now, let me simply re-emphasize that we need to use a great variety of foods in our basic approach to meals. If we have stressed anything in this book, we have stressed that many different chemical elements are needed by the body, and they work together in different combinations. We can only get what we need for the whole body if we include many different fruits, many different vegetables, many kinds of nuts and seeds, a variety of cereal grains, a little meat, different kinds of fish and poultry, a variety of herbal teas, and so on.

With this primary goal in mind, let's turn to some of the specific sexual problems that require special foods and attention.

A FEW WORDS ABOUT SPECIAL PROBLEMS

Of course impotence, sterility, sexually-transmitted diseases (STDs), and diseases like AIDS can be caused by infectious bacteria and viruses from outside the body. As we have seen, stress, depression, and chemical pollutants including alcohol, nicotine, and other drugs can also be responsible for sexual problems; in many cases the problem cannot be solved by dietary changes alone. In all instances of severe sexual problems both partners should seek the advice of a competent doctor.

Once a doctor has been consulted and it has been determined that causes of sterility, for example, are an unbalanced diet or poor lifestyle, the individual should consider fasting, sexual abstinence for one month, and then a balanced "building" diet based on my Master Feeding Program. Similarly, once functional causes of impotence have been considered and eliminated, you should realize that dietary deficiencies are a major part of the problem. Then a diet high in silicon, iron, and sulfur—and including such foods as whole grain cereals, seafood, onions, garlic, nuts, and

Special Foods and Recipes for the Sexual System

System Affected	Foods
Reproductive	Juices: blackberry, barberry, elderberry, cherry
Reproductive	Tonic of raw goat's milk with liquid chlorophyll, eucalyptus honey; raw egg yolk and clover honey in goat's milk; raw egg yolk in black cherry juice
Brain and Sex Center	Fish broth; onions, garlic, leeks, radishes; lean meat (from young animals only); Brussels sprouts, cauliflower, cabbage.
Stamina Center	Yogurt, cheeses; raw seed and nut butters; raw seed and nut milk drinks.

seeds—would be advised. (See chart above.) Women who suffer from ovarian and uterine problems (such as severe menstrual cramps and nausea, backaches, and lack of interest in sex) should first consult with their doctors. Here again, though, most women will find that my Master Feeding Program, along with warm drinks such as milk, elderberry juice, parsley tea, herbal tea with eucalyptus or white clover honey, will bring considerable relief. (See chart titled Foods for Ovarian Problems.)

LECITHIN

Lecithin is extremely important to our love lives. In men, it makes up 80 percent of the sex fluid. In both sexes, the brain is about 20 percent lecithin and 13 percent cholesterol, which make up the white matter or myeline coating of the nerves. Lecithin and cholesterol are needed by the endocrine glands. Lecithin affects the sex center of the brain, the transmission of nerve messages having to do with sexuality, and the endocrine glands. We must pay special attention to lecithin, and be very certain that our systems have enough to function properly.

What is lecithin made of? Classified as a phospholipid, lecithin is made of glycerol, fatty acids, phosphoric acid, inositol, and choline. Acetylcholine, a neurotransmitter involved in sexual arousal, may derive its choline from lecithin. Lecithin in the blood

Foods for Ovarian Problems

Warm honey drinks	Hot gruel
Elderberry juice	Rice water
Warm goat's milk	Broths
Parsley tea	Eggs
Fresh goat's milk with lemon juice	Black cohoch tea
Seed milk drinks	Dong quai

keeps cholesterol flowing, so that it doesn't deposit on artery walls as in arteriosclerosis.

I believe lechthin is often lacking in the American diet because it is so easily destroyed (by heating foods over 212°F.). Frying or scrambling eggs destroys the lecithin, so we need to boil or poach our eggs to get the most good out of them. Roasting soybeans, seeds, and nuts also destroys lecithin, as does the baking of whole grain breads.

The best lecithin for the brain is derived from animal products. The work of Dr. David Samuel in Israel found egg yolk lecithin superior to soy lecithin in restoring impaired memory and reducing withdrawal symptoms in addicts. Another excellent source of lecithin is raw fish roe (fish eggs) such as codfish roe, which can be found in the specialty food section of some markets or in delicatessens or gourmet food stores. Lecithin is also in meat, chicken, and fish, but remember cooking destroys it. Raw yogurt, raw goat milk, and cream are additional sources of lecithin.

Raw seed and nut butters are excellent sources of lecithin for all tissues of the body but the brain, nerves, and glands. (Every cell of the body needs lecithin.)

In a sense, the brain and sexual system in men compete for lecithin, creating a teeter-totter effect when either one is overused. Overuse of the brain not only causes brain fatigue but depletes lecithin from the sexual system as well. Overuse of the sexual system depletes brain lecithin, reducing motivation, creativity, our decision-making capacity and ability to think. There are rare individuals who combine genius, talent, and a sex life that would be excessive for most, but they have unusually strong metabolisms and exceptional constitutions.

How do we take lecithin? Try mixing a tablespoon of codfish roe (or any other roe) with a little tomato juice in a blender. A raw egg yolk in black cherry juice is a great tonic for the reproductive system, nerves, and brain. Soy lecithin has a mild tastes, and some people take a teaspoonful or tablespoonful and let it melt in their mouths. Lecithin can be mixed with almost any kind of juice in a blender. Also, I have found that vitamin E complements lecithin and increases its effectiveness.

PROGRAM FOR REVERSING INFERTILITY

If the condition blocking pregnancy is reversible, the program I describe here will often produce good results. Both partners must participate for best results, even if only one is known to have a problem with infertility.

The first step is to honestly confront the question of whether both partners really want to have a child, or whether one or both may fear having a child. Not wanting a child or fearing having a child can contribute to sterility in either partner. Fear of pregnancy is known to hinder or prevent pregnancy in a high percentage of infertile women.

Seeking professional counsel may help untangle psychological snarls. If a couple is not getting along properly, restoring harmony may also help restore fertility.

If the problem is not psychological, we move on to the physical level. Our initial objective is to make sure the body tissues of both partners are clean and rested. First, both partners should agree not to have sexual relations for a month while we are cleansing and resting all body systems. Second, both persons should participate in a tissue cleansing program, either by using my seven-day colema program or by going through a series of two limited periods of fasting (usually three days each). Both the colema program and various methods of fasting are described in my book, *Tissue Cleansing Through Bowel Management*. Supervision by a doctor is advised in either case.

During the 30 days of sexual abstinence, cleansing, and rest, we have two objectives. Over the first fifteen days, we want to get rid of potential blocks to fertility. Tobacco, alcohol, and drugs (except for necessary prescription drugs) should be avoided. The purpose of fasting or colemas is to get rid of toxic material stored in the body tissues. These toxins may be hindering fertility. The focus of the first fifteen days is on tissue cleansing. The focus of the last fifteen days is to build up all body systems with proper foods, exercise, attitudes, and rest.

The diet on nonfasting days will be my Master Feeding Program, with supplements as described later. I encourage the men not to wear jockey-type shorts but rather to wear boxer shorts for this period; and I ask the ladies not to wear all-nylon undergarments. Either can reduce fertility.

This thirty-day period should be very positive, very romantic, each partner being very supportive toward the other. Be as complimentary and considerate as possible. Arguments are against the doctor's orders. There can be no criticism, teasing, or mocking, no raising of the voice or lowering of the eyebrows, no pointing or game playing. Sincerity is necessary, as well as kindness, patience, acceptance, and friendliness.

After the tissue cleansing work, men should follow the Master Formula for Men; and the women should follow the Master Formula for Women, adding the supplements recommended for infertility.

In addition to taking my Master Formula, I want both men and women to take the following after each meal:

- 10 Sun Chlorella tablets, each meal
- 250 mg. vitamin C
- 1 tsp. cod liver oil
- 1 tsp. fresh bee pollen
- 1 tsp. sesame seed butter or tahini
- 1 juice glass aloe vera (may be mixed with fruit juice)
- Ginseng, according to directions on box or bottle

The following should be taken once daily:

- 1 tbsp. codfish roe (with tomato juice) or 1 raw egg yolk in black cherry or blackberry juice
- Lecithin
- 1 tbsp. rice bran syrup
- Nova Scotia dulse (flakes or liquid drops)
- Alfalfa sprouts
- Hawthorne Berry Tea
- Echinacea
- Oat straw tea
- Kyolic tablets

The rest of the Master Formula items for each sex should be taken as directed (usually three times daily). Herbs should be taken in the form of teas, but capsules may be used.

At the end of the thirty-day fertility restoration program, normal sexual relations may be resumed, but a celebration should be held to mark this as a special day.

I suggest that the couple plan a romantic day together, doing things that they both love to do. Go for a nature walk, ride horseback, or visit the beach. Have a romantic candlelight dinner and prepare for a leisurely, enjoyable time in the bedroom.

Many times, this thirty-day program is just the right ticket to overcome problems of infertility due to dietary deficiencies or toxic encumbrances in the body.

Now let's look at my Master Supplements and how to prepare them.

Chapter Twenty-Two
Master Supplements and Suggestions for a Super Sex Life

Many of the supplements discussed in this chapter will be new to you, and possibly some that you've been familiar with will have some surprises for you. This section should be a wonderful benefit to those whose sex lives have become routine, lackluster, or nonexistent, but even if your love life is already good, it should get better if you follow some of the suggestions presented here.

Keep in mind that special supplements to improve one's love life become less and less impressive the healthier you get because the healthier you get, the more enjoyable your life becomes. Many people are in such poor health that they will not get much good from the nutrients in my Master Formula until they have remained faithful to my Master Feeding Program for at least two months. It usually takes one year to make a significant difference in the quality of the tissue in our bodies.

The following Master Supplements have been particularly beneficial to me and to the people I have treated. I hope you agree that they add zest to your sex life.

Aloe Vera

Aloe Vera can be purchased at most health food stores or can be made from aloe plants grown in pots at home or in your yard. *Aloe barbadensis* is the scientific name for this thick-leaved, spiny-edged succulent plant from which the gel or juice is taken.

The healing properties of the aloe have been known for thousands of years, and the plant is mentioned in the Bible. It is used internally and externally. Because of its multiple effects and mildness, it may be classified as a tonic.

As far as the reproductive system is concerned, aloe vera juice (taken orally) is of great value in cleansing and soothing the internal organs—stomach, pancreas, liver, kidneys, lungs, glands, and so forth. Some people claim to feel warmth and tingling in specific internal areas after using aloe vera, calling it a pleasant sensation. The cleaner the body is internally, the more sensitive, potent, and active the reproductive system becomes.

Externally, aloe vera can be used on any rash or inflammation. It does not sting or burn. In fact, it soothes bee stings and burns. The juice can be diluted and used safely as a douche for vaginitis or leukorrhea, or (again diluted) can be used in an enema to relieve colitis.

Researchers say aloe vera contains as many as 75 biologically active ingredients including several B vitamins, choline and vitamin C, as well as calcium, chlorine, manganese, potassium, sodium and sulphur. Aloe vera has 18 amino acids, many plant sugars, natural "antibiotics" called anthra quimones that cleanse and relieve itching and reduce inflammation. It has at least five enzymes. Aloe vera also contains a potent fungicide that has proven effective against athlete's foot and many stubborn fungus infections.

If you want to make your own aloe vera tonic, I suggest two methods; one for internal use, the other for external application. Cut two large aloe leaves at the base of the plant, wash in water, and cut off the tip and spiny edges. For external application, cut into chunks, then mix in a blender. Apply full strength to the skin or dilute with water for a douche or enema. Do not take this internally because the outer skin can cause diarrhea when taken with the aloe gel. For internal use, take a sharp paring knife and trim two large aloe leaves as previously described, then slice them edgewise into very thin slices. Put the slices into a quart jar as soon as you have cut about a dozen, so you don't lose any of the gel. When both leaves are sliced and in the jar, add distilled water up to the top. Put a lid on the jar and refrigerate overnight. Stir in the morning, pour half a juice glass (liquid only—don't swallow the leaf sections) and add grape juice or orange juice to flavor. I like the natural taste, so you should try it to determine your preference. When you make the solution by soaking aloe vera slices, the green skin causes no problems. Take half a juice glass with each meal, and refill the quart jar (up to two times) when the liquid level is down to half full. Always let the juice soak for ten to twelve hours.

Many people use aloe vera as an internal tonic for a month, then skip two months, then take it a month and repeat the pattern.

Bee Pollen

Honeybee pollen has long been considered a sexual system vitalizer, probably because of its highly-concentrated collection of raw, pure nutrients. It is said to be the only nutritionally complete food known to man. Pollen is 20 percent protein and is also rich in fatty acids and carbohydrates. It is 15 percent lecithin, needed by the brain, nerves, and sexual system, and it contains natural plant steroids which are thought to nourish and stimulate the glands that produce our sex hormones. Loaded with all the major vitamins (and flavenoids) pollen contains a significant percentage of nucleic acids ("youth factors") and minerals such as calcium, phosphorus, iron, copper, sulfur, potassium, magnesium, manganese, silicon, sodium, iodine, zinc, and traces of other minerals. Keep in mind that pollen ingredients vary from area to area of the world, or even within the same country or state.

Research reports from the Soviet Union show that bee pollen has been successfully used to treat nervous and endocrine disorders. The Russians found that taking bee pollen increases recovery time after physical exertion (in athletes). While using pollen to successfully treat prostate problems in men, German and Swedish doctors found a hormone in bee pollen that stimulates the sex glands. There are many reports of pollen enhancing or restoring sexual vitality.

Pollen may be purchased at many health food stores, and sometimes directly from local beekeepers. It is best when fresh, since loss of nutrients is 75 percent in only a year. Try a teaspoon a day, or more if you choose. It tastes good plain or mixed with fruit juice.

Chlorella

Chlorella is an edible microalga grown under controlled conditions in large tanks in order to create one of the most powerful and beneficial nutrient sources known to man. It is sold in most health food stores in the form of small tablets, capsules, granules, or powder, and is generally taken as a supplement at meal times (five 200 mg. tablets with each meal).

Dr. Benjamin Frank has pointed out that our RNA and DNA production decreases with age, resulting in lower vitality, increasing incidence of ill health, and the common signs of aging. To counter this aging process, he recommended a diet high in foods containing RNA and DNA. With 10 percent RNA and three percent DNA, chlorella is one of the foremost "youth" nutrients known.

I have traveled to Japan and China to look into chlorella on my own, as described in my book *Chlorella: Gem of the Orient.* Allow me to share some of the knowledge I have learned about chlorella.

Chlorella is the highest known vegetable source of chlorophyll, nature's foremost cleanser, detoxifier and one of the best blood builders. It is also one of the highest vegetable sources of vitamin B-12, containing 70 percent of the recommended daily allowance in each three grams, the usual daily intake of chlorella.

I believe that chlorella is one of the greatest supplements in our time to restore or enhance the reproductive system because it cleanses, strengthens, and builds up every gland, organ, and tissue, every body system, so that the sexual system is naturally enhanced. This will make the body even more responsive to other nutrients, exercises, and processes taken to build up the sex life. For example, Chlorella cleanses the blood and lymph systems and helps build up the red blood cell count. It improves bowel elimination by feeding the bowel beneficial flora and stimulating peristaltic motion.

The liver is purified and strengthened in its many activities. Chlorella helps the body eliminate heavy metals, chemical pollutants, and drug residues. Chlorella's affinity for toxic chemical substances makes it an effective detoxifier and cleanser.

Cell repair throughout the body is stimulated and aided by the nucleic factors in chlorella. This includes the glands of the endocrine system, so important in human sexuality. Chlorella strengthens the body's natural immune system to protect against debilitating illness and disease. By reducing acidity in the body, chlorella soothes and protects the brain and nervous system.

In brief, chlorella tends to keep the body free of debilitating, energy-sapping substances and conditions so that we are free to enjoy our sexuality more fully.

The best available chlorella is Sun Chlorella, processed to break down the cell wall and increase the digestibility to 83 percent, more than any other available chlorella.

Chlorophyll

Because a body congested with catarrh, metabolic wastes, heavy metals, drug residues, chemical food additives, and air/water pollutants seldom feels like making love even when everything else in life is going well, we need to be concerned with keeping the insides of our bodies clean. Taking **chlorophyll** is one of the best ways of doing just that. Remember, a clean bloodstream is one of the biggest preliminary conditions for honest-to-goodness passion.

Chlorophyll, the pigment that makes plants green, is the most effective cleanser and detoxifier of the blood and lymph systems in nature. It also detoxifies the liver and builds up the beneficial bacterial in the bowel.

The chlorophyll molecule is identical to the hemoglobin molecule of the blood except for one difference: Chlorophyll has a magnesium atom at its center, while hemoglobin has an iron atom. This is why chlorophyll is such a great blood builder, since green plants contain iron in addition to all the other structured elements for making hemoglobin, the pigment that makes blood red.

The foods highest in chlorophyll are chlorella, spirulina, barley grass, wheat grass, parsley, and the leafy green vegetables. (The fiber in green vegetables helps keep the bowel toned and healthy as well as the chlorophyll.) Chlorella is 2.1 percent chlorophyll, spirulina is 0.8 percent, and alfalfa is 0.2 percent; commercial chlorophyll is usually derived from alfalfa. Liquid chlorophyll can be purchased at most health food stores, but the best way to get the chlorophyll you need is through plenty of salads and leafy green vegetables, supplemented by a concentrated chlorophyll as found in chlorella.

Dulse and Other Seaweed

I have been advising my patients to use Nova Scotia **dulse** for nearly fifty years because iodine is one of the most common deficiencies I encounter among those who come to me. Dulse is also rich in trace minerals, such as vanadium, chromium, bromine, lithium, fluoride, and vitamins A, B-complex, C, D, and K.

Dulse is one of several nourishing varieties of seaweed, which includes **Irish moss** and the many varieties of "**nori**" found in Oriental markets. All are rich in iodine, the chemical element needed to make the thyroid hormone. Kelp contains calcium, copper, boron, barium, strontium, and zinc as well as iodine and many vitamins.

The thyroid gland, by controlling the amount of thyroid hormone released into the bloodstream, determines the basic energy level of the body. It is also associated with the rate at which sex hormones are manufactured. Depression and loss of sex interest are often due to an underactive thyroid, which can be triggered by iodine deficiency.

A regular supplement of dulse or other seaweed is the best way to insure an adequate supply of iodine.

Garlic

According to an ancient manuscript discovered in East Turkistan, **garlic** was used as a health aid as early as 500 B.C. It is a natural antiseptic and germicide, a tonic to the lymph system, a cleanser and detoxifier for the lungs and liver, and a soothing relief to the bladder. Garlic balances the endocrine glands and helps restore balance during glandular disorders.

In the Caucasus and in Bulgaria men and women 100 years old or more chewed garlic for health and longevity. Many of these people were still sexually active. (Of course, garlic isn't the only reason, but it is one of the reasons!)

If you think the odor of garlic on your breath would ruin all the wonderful benefits, try taking Kyolic tablets, a form of high-quality deodorized garlic.

Herbs

Herbal preparations are milder, safer, and take longer to produce an observable effect than drugs. That's because they are foods, not medicines. But like foods, not all herbs may agree with everyone. Since many herbs produce similar effects, just avoid those that bother you.

The best way to take an herb is in the form of a tea made from the roots and bark (called a decoction) or leaves and blossoms (called an infusion). You can buy the raw ingredients from health food stores (and some supermarkets, depending on where you live). Alternatively, most health food stores sell herbs in capsule form to be taken orally. (You can break the capsules to make tea if you wish.) Tea is said to work better than swallowing the capsules.

Tea from roots or bark. If the herb is powdered, use one teaspoon; if cut in pieces, use one tablespoon. Bring one cup of water to a gentle boil in a stainless steel saucepan, add the herb, and let the tea boil for 30 minutes. Allow it to stand for five minutes or more and strain out the solid residue before drinking. Use 3, four-ounce cups per day.

Tea from leaves or blossoms. Bring one cup of water to a boil. Add one teaspoon of the powdered herb, remove from the heat, cover, and let steep for 15 minutes. Use 3, four-ounce cups per day.

It is best to take herbal preparations for three months, then cut the amount to one-half after that. (See chart that follows.)

Herbal Teas and Their Benefits

Black Cohosh	Helps normalize menstrual flow and relieve cramps; used in many female pelvic conditions, female problems, uterine difficulties; said to contain a natural estrogen.
Black Hawthorne	Tonic to female reproductive system, eases cramps, aids uterine congestion, inflammation, or leukorrhea.
Blessed Thistle	Can be used in place of black cohosh or black hawthorne for menstrual problems.
Cayenne	Can be added (in small amounts) to other herbs to stimulate their action.
Cloves	Mild support of reproductive system, both sexes.
Dong Quai	Helps almost every female problem; may cause enlargement of breasts, a change of life regulator.
Echinacea	Tonic for reproductive system, both sexes.
False Unicorn	Used most often for female infertility or menstrual irregularity; tones uterus.

Herbal Teas and Their Benefits (continued)

Fennel	Mild support of reproductive system, both sexes.
Fenugreek	Mild support of reproductive system, both sexes.
Fo-ti Tien	Endocrine gland rejuvenation and reproductive system tonic, females.
Ginseng	Whole body tonic; stimulates hormone production and balancing, both sexes. (See Ginseng under separate heading for fuller description.)
Gotu Kola	Properties similar to those of Fo-ti and Ginseng; tonic for improved brain function and memory; often taken with Ginseng (both sexes).
Licorice	Tones and stimulates female glands; contains a steroid-like compound; stimulates adrenal cortex to produce cortisone and aldosterone (females, usually). Can be used with ginseng and sarsaparilla, both sexes. (WARNING: DO NOT TAKE IF YOU HAVE HIGH BLOOD PRESSURE, UNLESS UNDER SUPERVISION OF DOCTOR OR NUTRITIONIST!)
Oat Straw	Nerve tonic, aids in overian and uterine disorders.
Red Raspberry	Strenghtens female reproductive system.
Safflower	Mild glandular support, both sexes.
Sarsaparilla	Contains hormone-like compounds beneficial for the sexual systems of both men and women.
Saw Palmetto	Helps balance hormone levels; tonic for glands, both sexes.
Slippery Elm	Mild glandular tonic, both sexes.
Squaw Vine	Relieves congested uterus and ovaries, reduces menstrual cramps, supports female reproductive system (females).

Lactobacillus Acidophilus

It isn't the most romantic thing in the world to point out that the quality of our sex lives depends a great deal on the cleanliness and tone of our bowel, but it is true. The more high-fiber foods we eat (up to a point, of course), the faster our bowel transit time becomes and the fewer problems we have, not only with bowel-related diseases, but with the level of blood cholesterol and the amount of toxins that are able to enter the blood and tissues from the bowel.

Lactobacillus acidophilus is one of several hundred micro-organisms that lives in the average bowel. Lactobacillus is a "friendly bacteria." There are many "unfriendly" organisms, but if we feed and encourage the "friendly" bacteria, we get rid of the harmful types. Lactobacillus is found in yogurt or can be taken in more concentrated liquid or capsule form. High chlorophyll foods feed and encourage the growth of lactobacillus, and chlorella stimulates it growth more than any other known food substance.

I encourage those just starting on the path to better health to purchase lactobacillus in your local health food store (buy the capsule form) and follow the directions on the bottle. Take chlorella at the same time.

Malva

Malva is a common herb in the United States and elsewhere in the world. The leaves are rich in pro-vitamin A (carotene), which is good for the glandular- and eliminative systems; and root infusions are reportedly good for urinary tract infections, the kidneys, and the bladder. The liquid from boiled leaves and roots helps speed up the baby's delivery time.

Basically, malva is a gentle herb which aids in keeping the genitourinary system free of inflammations and toxic wastes.

Royal Jelly

Royal jelly is said to prolong life, build the sex glands, and restore vitality more effectively than any other food. High in B vitamins, lecithin, and antibacterial substances, royal jelly also contains minerals such as iron, calcium, copper, potassium, sulfur, phosphorus, and silicon. Like bee pollen, royal jelly is another honeybee product. It is fed to the queen bee, who lays up to 10,000 eggs a day, working day and night, eating only royal jelly. As compared to the average worker bee who lives from 28 to 42 days, the queen bee lives five to six years. Royal jelly is partly derived from bee pollen, which is the reproductive material of plants. It contains hormone-like substances that support the glands and reproductive system.

Seeds and Nuts

Seeds and nuts contain all the life-factors necessary to reproduce new plants, which means they are capable of tremendous nutritional support of our reproductive systems. I classify seeds and nuts as survival foods.

The date seed is said to be one of the highest sources of a compound similar to the male hormone. Citrus seeds are said to be high in substances like the female hormones. Our male and female hormones are built from the life factors in these seeds—vitamin E, lecithin, calcium, silicon, enzymes, and fatty acids. Did you know that pumpkin seeds are a wonderful source of zinc for the male prostate gland? When the body is deprived of the nutrients needed to build healthy glands and nerves, our reproductive system is altered and diminished. We need to incorporate more seeds, nuts, and sprouts into our diets.

Health food stores often carry tahini and sometimes other seed and nut butters, but you can also make them yourself at home with a Champion juicer. Soak the raw seeds or raw hulled nuts overnight in apple or pineapple juice, then run them through the Champion juicer in the morning. If you make sesame butter, use the hulled sesame seeds.

Seed and nut milk drinks are also good. Soak a quarter cup of hulled sesame, pumpkin, or sunflower seeds, or shelled almonds, in apple or pineapple juice overnight, just as for the seed and nut butters. The next morning, put the quarter cup of seeds or nuts in a blender. For the liquid, you can use fruit or vegetable juice or just plain water. You may want to add carob powder, dates, or honey to the water for flavor. Blend until well-mixed, pour into a glass, and drink.

By including a variety of raw seeds, nuts, and sprouts in our diets, we can keep our glands happy, our nerves calm, and our brains active, alert, and well-fed. If these things are taken care of, our love lives are delightfully awakened.

Sprouts

Sprouts are especially valuable because they constitute a whole, pure, and natural food with all the factors contributing to life. They are rich in enzymes and low in calories. Sprouts contain significant amounts of calcium, iron, and zinc, some of the B-complex vitamins, and vitamin C.

The addition of sprouts to the diets of non-reproducing animals in a major urban zoo revitalized the once lethargic creatures, and many of them produced offspring after showing no interest in mating for several years.

Sprouts should be sprinkled on every green salad, but they may also be taken as a between-meal snack. Alfalfa and mung bean sprouts are best. However, you can sprout many of the legumes (garbanzos, for example) and others (melon, cucumber).

Wheat Germ and Wheat Germ Oil

Wheat germ is the heart of the wheat kernel. It is removed in the process of producing refined white flour, which leaves white flour nutritionally worthless. The wheat germ itself is highly concentrated in nutrients. It contains 24 grams of protein per half cup and is high in the B-complex vitamins, vitamin E, and iron. It is so high in phosphorus that it is necessary to take eight ounces of low-fat milk with it to prevent a calcium-phosphorus imbalance. Wheat germ contains traces of magnesium, manganese and calcium. **Wheat germ oil** is a concentrated source of fatty acids, high in natural vitamin E.

Both wheat germ and wheat germ oil should be kept in the refrigerator to prevent rancidity. A tablespoon after each meal provides over 60 mg. of vitamin E, six times the RDA for adult men and nearly eight times the RDA for adult women.

Whex

Whex is dehydrated goat milk whey, excellent for neutralizing excess acidity in the body, soothing irritated nerves and feelings, and for bringing calcium deposited in the joints back into solution. It is excellent for developing "friendly" bowel bacteria and aids in elimination.

Each 100 grams of Whex contains the following amounts of minerals:

Potassium	3,800 mg.		Phosphorus	288 mg.
Sodium	372 mg.		Calcium	102 mg.
Magnesium	73 mg.		Silicon	54 mg.

Whex also contains traces of boron, aluminum, manganese, iron, tin, lithium, copper, titanium, silver, strontium, and chromium.

Whex is helpful in all rheumatoid conditions, stiffness of the joints, muscle weakness, and acidic conditions. All systems of the body will benefit from this high potassium and sodium food.

Glandular Extracts

Glandular extracts (protomorphogens) are made from the raw organs of farm animals and are sold in health food stores as pills or capsules. They do not contain hormones. When glandular extracts such as testes or ovaries are taken, they stimulate an invigorating response to the corresponding human glands if there are problems of functional underactivity in our glands. In other words, if there is something wrong with our sex glands, glandular extracts may help. If there isn't anything wrong, the extract will be digested just like any other food, with no glandular stimulation and no side effects. Orally taken glandular extracts are harmless, except for occasional histaminic reactions (something like an allergic response) in those who have had a venereal disease, or other sex system problem (such as infection, tumor, or lesion).

According to Dr. Morton Walker, the benefits of using raw glandular extracts are much more powerful than simply eating the glandular tissue would be. Raw glandulars are refined nucleic acids which act like enzymes in that they are carried by the blood to specific organs that need help. Pituitary extract goes to the pituitary gland, thyroid extract goes to the thyroid, testicular extract goes to the testes—unless, as I said before, there is no problem in the target gland, in which case it is digested like any food. The glandular extract does not replace or build new glandular cells in us. Rather, it stimulates and aids our own bodies to build the new cells.

Glandular extracts available include those from the hypothalamus, pineal, pituitary, thyroid, adrenal, and prostate glands, as well as from the testes, uterus, placenta, and ovaries. Like any other supplement, raw glandulars will not be effective without a good diet, rest, and frequent exercise. Chapter Twenty-Three describes an exercise plan that almost anyone—regardless of their age or conditioning—can learn to live with.

Chapter Twenty-Three
Exercises You Can Live With

Exercise helps reverse an unhealthy sex life, improve a so-so sex life, and enhance even a good sex life, provided that a few common-sense rules are followed.

The good news about exercise is that it helps keep our weight down, tones the muscles, strengthens the heart, reduces the risk of cardiovascular disease, keeps the joints working smoothly, moves the lymph through its circulatory system, and aids in getting blood circulation to the extremities, especially the head and brain. Exercise keeps the nerves sensitive, so that sex is more enjoyable, and reduces the effects of stress, which tends to reduce both the sex drive and enjoyment.

The bad news about exercise is that like any good thing, it can be overdone. Studies have shown, for example, that long-distance running or jogging is often accompanied by a reduced sex drive. Dr. Angelo Belcastro of the University of Alberta in Edmonton, Canada, said that men who run more than forty miles a week may be burning off hormones as fast as they are burning calories. They may suffer up to a complete loss of their sex drive. The same problem can occur with body building or prolonged aerobic exercise unless the hormone loss is compensated for by some means, such as nutritional and supplemental support.

Obviously, exercise may not be of much benefit unless it is accompanied by a properly-balanced food regimen and sufficient rest. This book provides guidelines for all three.

Some years ago, I met a man at a body-building center whose eyes were dark pits in his head and whose skin seemed a little loose over an otherwise well-muscled body. "What have you been doing?" I asked. "I've lost over 100 pounds this month by dieting, working out with weights each day, and sitting in the steam room for an hour," he replied. I wondered if the man had possibly shortened his life span by ten or fifteen years by putting his body and brain through such torture! This is greatly overdoing it.

If you exercise consistently and eat properly, you will lose weight if you are overweight. I have good news, very good news, for those who are overweight. As your weight comes down from right eating and sensible exercise, your sex drive is considerably enhanced. Apparently, obesity hinders the production of hormones that stimulate the sex drive in both men and women and reduces the sensory nerve stimulation that records sexual pleasure. To lower weight and keep it off, don't try to lose more than one pound each week.

WHAT KIND OF EXERCISE IS BEST?

The kind of exercise that's best for you will depend on your age, physical condition, personality type, and motivation. To a lesser degree, it will depend upon your available time, finances, and the facilities available in your area.

Some people play racquetball for an hour three times a week, a highly-competitive, physically-demanding exercise. It's great for people in good physical shape who don't like noncompetitive sports or exercise. Tennis and handball are, similarly, good exercise for competitors. Volleyball is sometimes okay, but the acceptability of team sports depends upon the consistency with which a person brings up his or her heart rate and breathing to a certain useful point for half an hour or so. Soccer and basketball are excellent because of the constant running involved. Baseball and softball, with their sitting in the dugout between innings and waiting for something to happen, might be fun but will not accomplish much for your conditioning. Neither will riding in a golf cart.

The problem with competitive sports is their irregularity for those of us who play only for pleasure, competition, and/or health benefits. Unless exercise can be regularly scheduled everyday for half an hour or three to four times a week for an hour every other day, it isn't really health enhancing.

Strenuous exercise is for young people—the "Under 40" crowd. If you are over 40 and want to stay in intensely competitive and strenuous sports, talk it over with your doctor first.

The best overall exercises are walking and swimming, half an hour each day. If you can't do either of those, here are some exercises, treatments, and tips to keep you at your healthy best.

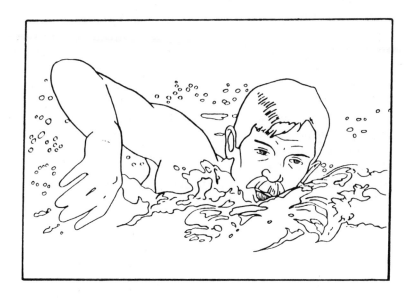

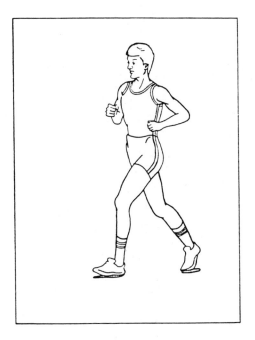

The Best Overall Exercises:

Swimming and Walking

My Bouncer Exercises

A "bouncer" is one type of mini-trampoline so popular these days. There are three great advantages to bouncer exercises. One is that you can do them to music of your choice to make the exercise more enjoyable. Another is that they can be done indoors (on rainy days). Another is that bouncer exercises don't have the "body shock" effect on the bones and joints that running and jogging have.

Here are some of my favorites.

For the easier-going crowd—those who are older, over-weight, or out of shape—here are some bouncer exercises especially for you, but talk to your doctor before you get into any exercise routine. Get his advice on your needs and limitations.

Hands and Arms Flex and More: Hold your arms out straight in front of you to start with, then flex your fingers and hands as you move your arms in time with the music, over your head, out to your sides, front.

Toes and Ankles: Lift up on the toes, swing heels toward and away from one another, then bring heels down and swing the knees in circles to the right, then to the left.

Knees: As you do the preceding, flex your knees without moving your feet from the bouncer, gently jogging.

Swimming: Make overhead swimming motions with your arms as you bounce gently to the music.

Hula Bounce: Move your hips, hula style, in circles, then side-to-side, front-to-back (thrusting and drawing back the pelvis) several times. Move arms and hands gracefully.

Shoulder Rolls: Rotate shoulders (with hands at sides) alternatively, left and right shoulder, forward circles, backward circles, then both shoulders. Keep legs moving and knees flexing.

Twist and Bend: Twist the body from side to side several times, bend forward, bend backward. Repeat, ten times.

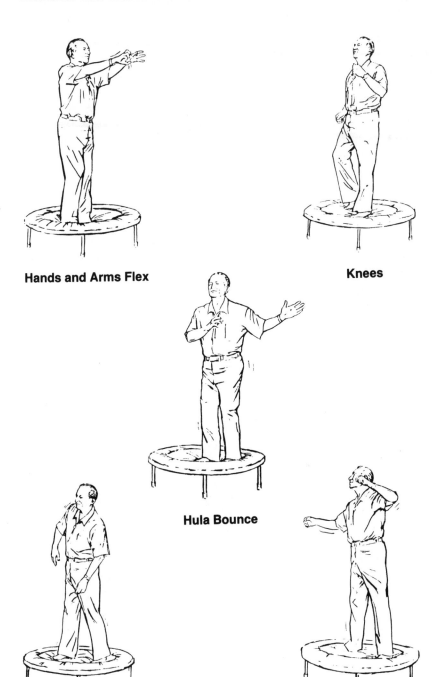

Hands and Arms Flex

Knees

Hula Bounce

Shoulder Rolls

Twist and Bend

Neck Exercise: Move the neck with movements like a Persian dancer. Rotate hips in circles, the knees and the arms also in circles.

Look ahead to the next section's Figure 8 exercises and do them on the bouncer. Start with shoulder and arm movements like Fred Astaire or Ginger Rogers in their classic dance films, as below.

Knee Crossing: Cross the right knee over the left, then the left knee over the right, as shown, six times. Change to the Charleston dance, and do it six times with small steps. (If you don't know how, ask your mother or grandmother to show you.)

Just for Kicks: Kick one foot forward, then the other, reaching down toward the toes of your kicking foot.

Elephant: Clasp hands in front of yourself, bend over with feet apart, knees straight, and stretch-swing your arms to the left then to the right as an elephant swings its trunk.

High Bounces: When you are used to the bouncer, get up in the air, improvise, do your own thing but keep in motion, that's the idea!

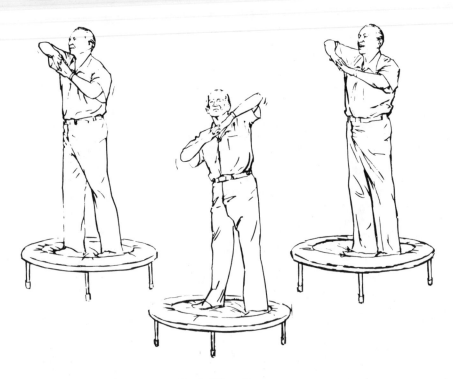

Neck Exercises

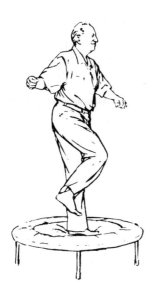

Knee Crossing

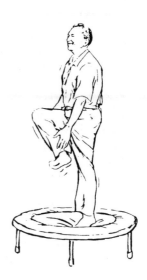

Just for Kicks

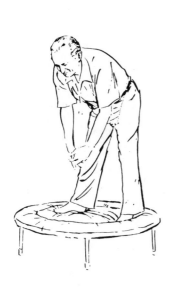

Elephant

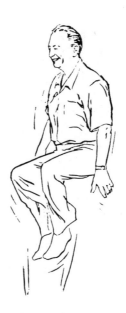

High Bounces

"Figure 8" Exercises

They say, "We're as young as our joints," because you need limber joints to do the things young people do. Figure 8 exercises are designed for the joints and follow the circular "8" pattern for maximum benefit.

Knee Joints Figure 8s: Put hands on knees and do Figure 8 circles ten times in each direction.

Hip Joints Figure 8s: Feet six to eight inches apart, swing hips and buttocks in a large Figure 8 pattern eight times in each direction.

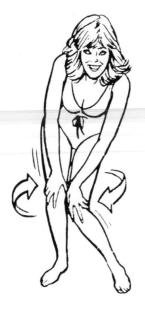

Knee Joints Figure 8s

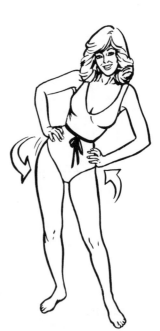

Hip Joints Figure 8s

Shoulder 8s: Visualize a Figure 8 around your shoulders, clasp arms, lead first with right shoulder, then left, ten times each.

Neck Figure 8s: Look straight ahead, try to make Figure 8s with your head, moving the neck only, as in Persian dancer movements previously described.

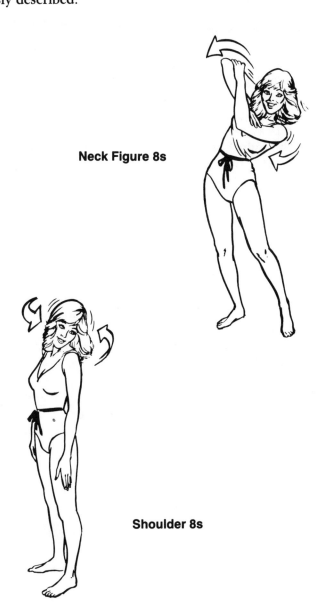

Neck Figure 8s

Shoulder 8s

Slanting Board Exercises

The primary purposes of slanting board exercises are to bring blood to the brain, to "tune up" the brain centers, to remove any pelvic pressure due to a prolapsed colon, and to tone the abdominal and pelvic organs. Be careful and take it easy at first.

1. Lie full length, allowing gravity to help the abdominal organs into their position. Lie on board for at least ten minutes.
2. While lying flat on your back, stretch the abdomen by putting arms above the head. Bring arms above the head ten to fifteen times. This stretches the abdominal muscles and pulls the abdomen down toward the shoulders.
3. Bring abdominal organs toward your shoulders while holding breath. Move the organs back and forth by drawing them upward, contracting the abdominal muscles, then allowing them to go back to a relaxed position.
4. Pat abdomen vigorously with open hands. Lean to one side then to the other, patting the stretched side. Pat ten to fifteen times on each side. Bring the body to a sitting position, using the abdominal muscles. Return to a lying position. Do this three to four times, if possible. Do only if doctor orders.
5. Bend knees at the hips. While in this position, (a) turn head from side to side five to six times; (b) lift head slightly and rotate in circles three or four times.
6. Lift legs to vertical position, rotate outward in circles eight or ten times. Increase to twenty-five times after a week or two of exercising.
7. Bring the legs straight up to a vertical position and lower them to the board slowly. Repeat three or four times. .
8. Bicycle legs in air fifteen to twenty-five times.

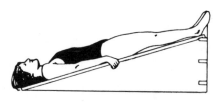

Figure 1

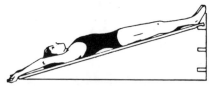

Figure 2

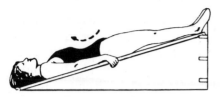

Figure 3

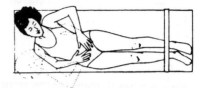

Figure 4

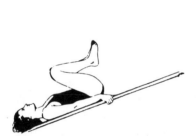

Figure 5

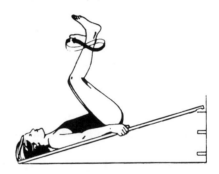

Figure 6

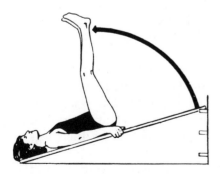

Figure 7

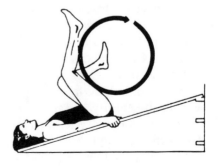

Figure 8

Skin Brushing

The skin gets rid of a good deal of toxic material each day, and, in so doing, reduces the amount that could otherwise be circulated in the blood and lymph and deposited in inherently weak tissues. It is necessary and helpful to remove the old skin cells by brushing with a long-handled, soft natural bristle brush to keep the pores open and free to eliminate wastes. Skin brushing stimulates the surface blood capillaries under the skin and helps keep the body clean.

Skin brushing should be done twice a day, morning and evening, before taking a bath or shower. Brush all areas of the body except the face, nipples, and sexual parts.

How to Improve Circulation

Besides the slant board, which aids in getting blood to the head, and exercises such as walking or swimming, there are several ways to get the blood moving throughout the body. These include the Kneipp water treatments, barefoot walks in sand or grass, and taking 100 mg. or more of niacin after each meal. No matter how well we are eating, it does us little good if the nutrients are not being transported by the blood and lymph to the tissues where they are needed.

Kneipp Water Treatment and Barefoot Walks

I once visited Worishofen, Germany, where Father Sebastian Kneipp developed and used the water cure. Father Kneipp had earlier cured himself of tuberculosis when doctors had given up on him, and he decided to devote his life to sharing the health discovery he had made.

Father Kneipp believed that cold water was live water and hot water was dead water. His baths in Worishofen were places where people could wade in cold water up to the groin. The water was so cold they really had to move because they wanted to complete their walk through the bath and get out. Then they let their legs dry in the open air.

If you don't have a place where you can wade groin-deep in cold water, take a water hose without a spray attachment and, starting from the toes, go up the right leg to the groin, then around and down the back of the right leg. Repeat on the left leg.

Do not dry yourself with a towel. Instead, walk barefoot in sand (as on a beach) or on grass (as in a park or on a lawn) until your legs and feet are dry, about 10 minutes. Be careful of where you are walking barefoot, especially if you have cuts on your feet or if the climate in your area is cold.

Do this exercise only once a day, and it will do wonders for your circulation.

The Niacin Flush

By taking niacin, 100 mg. or more with your meals, your skin will experience a reddening, flushing effect that signals blood is being brought to the face, scalp, and often to the torso and legs. The tingling or heat-effect is produced by the histamines that rush to the skin area at niacin's prompting. These sensations are harmless, but may be unpleasant to some.

Niacinamide will not do the job. It doesn't move the blood or flush the skin like niacin does. Niacin not only helps cleanse the body and move the blood but has other useful qualities as a vitamin.

Exercise for the Prostate Gland

In China many years ago I learned a wonderful exercise for the prostate gland which is said to be helpful in stimulating blood and lymph flow to the prostate. This exercise should help almost any prostate condition, and reportedly it brings dramatic relief in many cases of congestive prostatitis. If a man does not yet have prostate problems, I believe daily use of this exercise may prevent them from appearing.

Here's how the exercise is done. Stand up, feet together. Bend the knees until you're about one-third down in a squatting position. Now bring one knee forward, the other back, without moving the feet or lifting the heels. To increase the effectiveness of this exercise, try squeezing the buttocks together.

Continue moving the knees back and forth alternatively and rotating the pelvis forward on the same side where the knee is brought forward. Start with fifteen "knee-moves" back and forward with each knee the first week, then do two sets the second week (morning and evening).

Gradually increase the time taken for this exercise to ten minutes or more daily, preferably five minutes twice a day. This exercise, as you may guess, is a form of prostate "massage" that keeps the glandular tissue well-toned and healthy.

Kegel Exercise for the Ladies

For many years now, doctors have recognized that lack of enjoyment of lovemaking by the ladies was often correlated with flaccid or "out-of-shape" musculature around the vagina.

This exercise was developed by a doctor to restore muscle tone in the pubo-coccygeus muscle. Over the years it has been demonstrated to be very effective and successful in restoring and enhancing the love lives of those who practice it faithfully for several weeks.

The object is simply, during urination, to try to stop and start, stop and start, stop and start. When you can feel which muscle you're using, you don't have to restrict practice only to the times while you're urinating. You can practice anytime, anywhere.

Do this squeezing/relaxing exercise twenty times in the morning, at mid-day, and in the afternoon or evening. You can decide for yourself when you have reached a point where your muscular tone is sufficient.

EXERCISE IS SEXERCISE

Physically fit men and women seem to enjoy sex more than others, and I don't think this is mere illusion. When you exercise regularly, everything in your body works better, including your sexual system and the sensory nerves that relay pleasurable sensations to the brain.

Exercise and a good, balanced food regimen belong together. Most of us have been taught in school that exercise makes digestion and assimilation more efficient, so we get more good from our foods. Not as many of us know that exercise fights depression and favors a more pleasant disposition.

The brain, nerves, glands, and circulation of blood and lymph all benefit from exercise—and all of these are necessary for an active, enjoyable sex life. On the other hand, those who seldom if ever exercise tend to grow flabby, less energetic, less attractive, and experience more problems with their love lives.

Epilogue

To smile and mean it, you must have the right physio-chemical structure in your body, and that comes with proper diet, exercise, and lifestyle. I hope you now understand that no food regimen and exercise program, no matter how wonderful and complete, can ever cause you to have a better love life. You have to make up your mind first. Remember, the body always follows the mind.

Sexual desire has its root, proportion, and place in the soul life as the heart's yearning for completeness; while the sex drive has its root, proportion, and place in the physical life as nature's way of continuing the next generation. The degree to which you enjoy making love depends primarily upon the mind, but as we have seen, we can't really separate mind from body. Therefore, the better and more positive your thoughts and attitudes are about your mate and your sex life, the more you'll enjoy times of intimacy together. The mind initiates, the body responds.

On the other hand, we must acknowledge that the body and mind are designed to work best when all the right chemical elements are in all the right places in the body, and every physical system—the nervous, digestive, eliminative, circulatory, glandular, skeletal, and muscular systems—have everything they need to work right.

You can't really reach the place of expressing great love and of experiencing great sexual enjoyment and satisfaction until your life is working right and feeling great. For that to happen, you need to have body, mind, and spirit in harmony. A healthy body is a basic necessity in this process.

You can give a starving person a candy bar, and it will taste delicious. But it will ultimately deplete vitamins, minerals, and energy and leave the body in worse shape than before. The same is true of sex. You can have an unhealthy body and enjoy sex, but it will deplete your energy and enjoyment of life later on. Sex for a person in good physical condition, on the other hand, can increase alertness, enhance the mental faculties, cheer the heart and spirit, and put a twinkle in the eye and bounce in the step.

Great sex helps keep a person young and joyful!

When we get down to the bottom line, the process of working for better health and a better love life will elevate and express your soul life, your purpose on this planet. Great sex can help set a person free to express his or her purpose in life, but we must understand that sex can only become great when the quality of our relationship with our mate is at the highest possible level.

Proper nutrition, regular exercise, and a healthy lifestyle, as described in this book, will change not only your love life but your whole life!

This book is your guidebook, pointing the way to a higher path, joy in your relationships, and a better world. I wish you a lovely and productive "Bon voyage!"

Index

If You've Enjoyed Reading This Book . . .

. . . why not tell a friend about it? If you're interested in learning more about Dr. Bernard Jensen's approach to health, here are some other titles you may find to be informative, engaging, and fun.

Vibrant Health From Your Kitchen

A warm and wonderful tour through Dr. Jensen's latest discoveries about food, nutrition, and health, this book provides the guidance needed to keep your family disease-free, healthy, and happy.

Tissue Cleansing Through Bowel Management

Toxin-laden tissue can become a breeding ground for disease. This remarkable book instructs you in the removal of toxins and the restoration of health and youthfulness through the cleansing and care of the organs of elimination.

Food Healing for Man

We now know that foods can repair the tissue damage that accompanies most illness and disease. Look over the shoulders of the great pioneer nutritionists as they investigate the links between nutrition and disease.

Chlorella: Gem of the Orient

Why does Dr. Jensen consider chlorella—a green alga—the most valuable broad-spectrum food supplement discovery of the twentieth century? You'll find out in this unusually beautiful, fully illustrated, hard cover book.

Creating a Magic Kitchen

This is Dr. Jensen's introductory primer on the art of selecting and preparing foods for the best of health. Short, easy to understand, and handy to use, this is the perfect book for anyone who wants a more healthful and enjoyable lifestyle.

Nature Has a Remedy

This popular classic provides a delightful description of the many paths to natural healing—foods, herbs, exercise, climate selection, personology, and hundreds of effective remedies.

World Keys to Health and Long Life

Based on Dr. Jensen's travels to over fifty-five countries, this fascinating book describes the health and longevity secrets of centenarians interviewed in the Hunza Valley of India; Vilcabamba, Peru; the Caucasus Mountains of the Soviet Union; and other places around the world.

Doctor-Patient Handbook

Discover the reversal process and healing crisis that Nature uses to rid the body of disease and restore well-being. Here is a fresh approach to wholistic health.

Slender Me Naturally

Dr. Jensen's answer to fad diets that don't work is a natural weight loss program that does. Developed over fifty-eight years of experience with overweight patients, this program is a healthful and effective way of losing unwanted weight.

Breathe Again Naturally

Get rid of asthma, allergies, bronchitis, hay fever, and other respiratory problems. Dr. Jensen discusses nutrition, herbs that work, food supplements, breathing exercises, attitude, and climate.

Arthritis, Rheumatism and Osteoporosis

Are you among the one in four Americans who suffers from arthritis, rheumatism, or osteoporosis? Would you like to know what to do about it? This book is for you.

Foods That Heal

This book presents the basic principles of Hippocrates, Dr. Rocine, and Dr. Jensen regarding the use of foods to help the body regain health. The author has also included a complete guide to the various fruits and vegetables we all need.

In Search of Shangri-La

Here is the very personal journal of Dr. Jensen's physical and spiritual travels through China into Tibet, and his reflections on his search for Shangri-La.

Beyond Basic Health

Dr. Jensen looks at the deteriorating state of modern man's health and offers practical advice and insights to those health professionals who must deal with today's devastating illnesses.

For information regarding prices, write to:

Hidden Valley Health Ranch
Route 1 Box 52
Escondido, California 92025